nutrition

in essence

Sarah Bearden

Series Editor: Nicola Jenkins

Hodder Arnold

A MEMBER OF THE HODDER HEADLINE GROUP

Orders: please contact Bookpoint Ltd, 130 Milton Park, Abingdon, Oxon OX14 4SB. Telephone: (44) 01235 827720. Fax: (44) 01235 400454. Lines are open from 9.00 - 5.00, Monday to Saturday, with a 24 hour message answering service. You can also order through our website www.hoddereducation.co.uk

If you have any comments to make about this, or any of our other titles, please send them to educationenquiries@hodder.co.uk

British Library Cataloguing in Publication Data
A catalogue record for this title is available from the British Library

ISBN-10: 0 340 92730 5
ISBN-13: 978 0 340 92730 4

This Edition Published 2006
Impression number   10 9 8 7 6 5 4 3 2 1
Year   2010   2009   2008   2007   2006

Hodder Headline's policy is to use papers that are natural, renewable and recyclable products and made from wood grown in sustainable forests. The logging and manufacturing processes are expected to conform to the environmental regulations of the country of origin.

The information given in this book is not intended as a replacement for medical advice and should not be used for diagnosis or treatment of any medical condition.

Cover photo from Ryan McVay/Photodisc Green/Getty Images

Typeset by Servis Filmsetting Ltd, Manchester
Printed in Great Britain by CPI Bath

acknowledgements

This book could not have been written without the support of the following people:

Those at Hodder Arnold, who turned my manuscript into this beautiful book - you include Nicola Jenkins, Tamsin Smith, Claire Baranowski and Lyn Ward, as well as others behind the scenes. A special thanks to Nicola Jenkins for her professionalism, support and friendship.

I would also like to thank my teachers along the way, especially Lawrence G. Plaskett, PhD., and Paula Bartholomy, M.S.

A very special thank you is extended towards Rebecca Katz, 'The Inner Cook', who helped me tremendously with recipe development. Thank you's also go to those friends and colleagues for their expertise, love and support. I have bounced nutrition ideas off of all of you for years and you graciously put up with me. You include Jennie Harding, Willie Victor, JJ Virgin, Rebecca Katz, Donna Shoemaker, Tiffany Brine ("Little Sis"), Jaya Schillinger, Jodi Weitz, Connie Prodromou, Marianne Rogoff, Meredith Mill, Dave Woodgate, Emma Backshall and Russell Jackman, who kept my computer humming and happy.

This book is dedicated with great love to my family: David, Holly and Tim Bearden. You really do light up my life. This book is also dedicated in memory of my father, Arleigh D. Richardson III: my first and best teacher.

The author and publishers would like to thank the following for the use of photographs in this volume:

p5, 30 ABPL/Maximilian, p6 © photocuisine/Corbis, p7–9, 16, 17, 36, 37, 39 (top), 43, 48, 59, 68, 82, 87, 89, 93, 96, 111, 114, 121–123 PurestockX, p21 Sam Bailey, p26, 125 Carl Drury, p27, 58 © Royalty-Free/Corbis, p39 (bottom) Maximilian Stock Ltd/Jupiterimages, p49, p56 ABPL/Joy Skipper, p50 © istockphoto.com/Mikhail Tolstoy, p86 Ingram, p100 © dk/Alamy, p124 plainpicture GmbH & Co KG/Photolibrary

v

326362

contents

nutrition – the basics

Nutrition is a very confusing topic for most people these days. If you pick up a woman's magazine or watch any morning television programme you are likely to find that an article or presentation about nutrition is trying to convince you that a particular fad diet, or a particular group of nutrients, will be the one secret that positively changes your life forever. Yet, the more you read magazine articles or watch television shows, the more you are likely to be in the dark as to which advice to follow, because many of them are contradictory. How can this be so? A fad diet is often presented by someone who found a diet that worked for them and they wish to share this diet with the world. Unfortunately, the secret of magic nutrients is that there is usually a product for sale behind the hype.

Nutrition in Essence does not advocate any particular dietary philosophy, nor does it tell you what to do. You won't find any fad diets here. What you *will* find are the dietary guidelines that have proved to be of greatest benefit for those people who wanted to increase their energy, to feel and look vibrant and to be the healthiest they can be. The bonus is that as you read these guidelines you will see that the underlying theme is a focus on foods that are absolutely delicious. Practising the art of nourishment is not one of sacrifice. You may be happily surprised to learn that some foods that you've been told are bad for you are actually good for you!

Common sense would tell you that in order to achieve health through diet it would be best to consume foods that are close to what Nature has provided for you. After all, the way your body works is not that different from the way your caveperson ancestor's body worked, when the only food available was wild game and plant foods. Luckily, you don't have to forage for your food like your ancient ancestor, but the same principles of nutrition that worked for your ancestors will also work for you.

This book advocates that a diet primarily consisting of wholefoods is the healthiest diet for anyone to follow. However, the term 'wholefoods' is a very general one, and the individual foods chosen will vary from person to person, according to their individual needs. This approach allows for the recognition of a term that a biochemist named Roger Williams used back in the 1950s: the concept of biochemical individuality. Biochemical individuality may not sound very romantic,

but it acknowledges that every one of us is unique in our nutritional needs. This approach to diet also explains why some diets work for some people, but don't work for others. Once you have mastered the definition of what wholefoods are and you have read about the different health issues covered in this book, you will be able to craft a diet that is right for you as an individual. You will be able to choose the foods that nourish you the best, avoid the ones that may be problem foods for you and select the foods that you actually like to eat. Isn't this more fun than having someone tell you what to do and following a diet that is full of foods that you don't even like? The 'In a nutshell' sections in this book include recipes and cooking techniques that show how delicious wholefoods are and how easy they are to prepare.

If what you have read so far appeals to you, you will want to find out more about the essence of good nutrition. Let's start with some definitions of terms.

What are wholefoods?

Since *Nutrition in Essence* advocates the use of wholefoods, let's become clear about what we mean by this term. Here is a definition:

Wholefoods are the edible parts of foods that are as close to their natural state as possible and are prepared in a way that retains enough nutritional value to be supportive of health.

Using this definition, it is obvious that an apple, a carrot and a bunch of leafy greens are wholefoods, because they can be picked and eaten in their natural state. If you consider the example of the apple, you know that the edible part of the apple is most of the apple itself, but you probably would not eat the core and the seeds. However, apple juice is not a wholefood. To make the juice, you need many apples, which are processed through a juicer. The juice is extracted and then the fibre is thrown away. The juice, though high in vitamins, will also be high in sugar because the natural fibre which would have slowed down the digestion of this sugar is gone. High amounts of sugar are not supportive to health. Therefore, a glass of apple juice is not as healthy a choice as a whole apple would be.

Cooked or raw?

Some people ask if eating a wholefood diet means that all food needs to be raw. This is not the case. Certainly, there are many foods that can be eaten raw (such as the apple), but a puréed leek and potato soup would be a wholefood meal because you started with leeks and potatoes in their natural state and they remained in their natural state as wholefoods before you cooked and blended them. They may have lost a few vitamins through cooking, but they still retain most of their nutrient value – enough to be supportive of health. Even though they have been cooked and blended, they are still wholefoods.

Some foods should never be eaten raw. For example, cashew nuts are heated during their extraction from their shells in order to remove a caustic resin that exists between the nut and its shell. This is why you won't find cashews in their shells in stores.

Certain nutrients in foods are actually enhanced by being cooked; the phytonutrient lycopene found in tomatoes is found in greater amounts in cooked tomatoes than in raw tomatoes. Tomatoes are also a good source of vitamin C and this vitamin is vulnerable to heat. So tomatoes are wholefoods which 'retain enough nutritional value to be supportive of health' in both their raw and cooked forms.

Some people ask if a food like tofu is a wholefood because they have read that it is a healthy food. In this case it is not a wholefood, because to make tofu you have to separate out parts of the soya bean and throw parts of it away. What about boxed wholegrain flaked cereal from the health food store; is that a wholefood? No, because cereals like this have first been made into slurries, heated to high temperatures and have often had synthetic nutrients added to them. Using our definition of wholefoods, these cereals are pretty far away from their natural state and it is debatable as to whether their nutritional value is supportive of health. If you read the nutrition labels on the box, you will find that manufactured cereals are often full of sugar (even though the sugar in them is often touted as 'natural') and the fibre content is not really the same as it would be if you were eating the wholegrain.

Can a wholefood be processed? Yes: if you take whole wheat berries and grind them into a wholemeal flour, this is a form of processing, but you still have all the original parts of the wheat berries.

What are refined foods?

Refined foods are those foods which have been processed so that most of their nutrients have been stripped away from them. So, for example, white rice is refined, while brown rice is not. Many of the boxed and packaged foods you find in your supermarket have refined foods in them. Refined foods can also be processed foods. Refined foods are actually nutrient thieves because in addition to not providing nutrients they actually rob your body of stored nutrients in order to make the energy it takes to digest them. If you live on a diet of refined foods, you can become depleted of the nutrients you need.

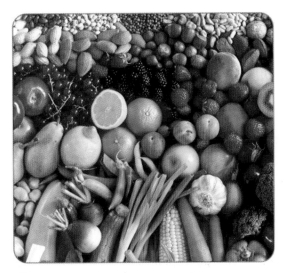

A plant-based diet

Is a plant-based diet vegetarian or vegan? It can be, but it doesn't have to be. Plant-based means that most of your food comes from plants and not animal products. You can eat a variety of meat, poultry and seafood and still have a plant-based diet. If you imagine a dinner plate and more than half of that plate has foods that come from plants, this is a plant-based meal.

In each chapter of *Nutrition in Essence*, you will see that you are recommended to follow the 'Guidelines for a healthier diet'. The guidelines are listed below. If you plan to follow them, we do not expect you to make drastic changes in your current diet. As you learn more about healthy foods, you may want to begin by gradually incorporating these guidelines in your menu planning. At first, you may need to spend some time finding out where you can buy your wholefoods. You may wish to incorporate more wholefoods into your diet gradually. Therefore these guidelines are preceded by the phrase 'as much as possible'.

General guidelines for a healthier diet
   As much as possible:

- Incorporate wholefoods into your diet.
- Choose organic foods.
- Eat a plant-based diet. (Refer to the definition above.)
- If you shop in a supermarket, buy food from the outside aisles (e.g. fruit and vegetables). This is where you will find most of the fresh wholefoods.
- Eat foods that are locally grown and in season.
- Avoid sugar and refined foods.
- Eliminate bad fats from your diet and replace them with good fats.
- Limit irritating substances such as caffeine and alcohol and replace some of your consumption of these with water, herb teas and nutrient-rich broths such as 'Vital Vegetable Broth' (Recipe on p. 11). Make sure you are hydrated.

- ℔ Avoid using artificial sweeteners. They are loaded with chemicals and have no place in a wholefood diet.
- ℔ Use portion control and do not skip meals.
- ℔ Try not to eat the same foods over and over every day.
- ℔ Try to follow the suggestions given in 'Specifics of a wholefood diet' (see below).

Specifics of a wholefood diet: wholefoods and wholefood helpers

Let's look at individual food categories so that you will have a better idea of what kinds of foods we are recommending. This list includes all categories of foods, including animal foods. If you are a vegetarian or vegan, just focus on the recommendations that are plant-based. The preparation methods suggested are those which best help to conserve the nutrients of the foods.

Meat and seafood

Meat is often maligned in nutrition books. This is unfair. It is the source and the quality of the meat and the amount of meat consumed that are important. Sadly, most of today's meat is raised on factory farms where the animals are grown in cruel, crowded conditions and they are given antibiotics and growth hormones. They are given feed that is not organic, which is not what they would naturally be eating if they were grazing as they were meant to do. But these are totally different animals from animals grown on organic, sustainable farms where good farming is practised. These animals are free-range and grass-fed, as they should be. This source of meat is healthy. Similarly, many of the fish we buy are from fish farms. These fish are raised on feed and are also given

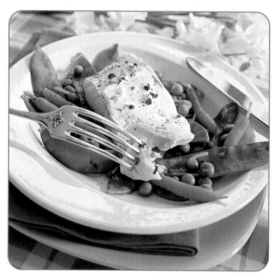

Meat and fish can be part of a healthy diet but should be eaten in moderation

antibiotics. In the wild, fish naturally eat algae and other micro-organisms they find for themselves. These are the fish that are high in essential fats. Meat and poultry that are organic and pasture-raised or fish caught in the wild will be the healthiest choices. The fats and protein of fish and red meat are healthiest if the food is just cooked through (not charred), though poultry and pork should always be well cooked.

Dairy

Many people have a difficult time with dairy, but this is often because dairy is highly processed. Pasteurised milk is difficult to digest because the protein of the milk has been damaged due to high heat. If you can find organic raw milk and raw cheese, this actually can be very health beneficial. Often, people who think they are sensitive to dairy find they do well on raw dairy products. Many indigenous cultures around the world consume dairy and are healthy and they consume it raw. Some people find that they are sensitive to cow dairy but can well tolerate goat and sheep dairy. You can read more about food intolerances in Chapter 11.

Eggs

Eggs are very healthy foods. However, they should come from chickens that are free range and grass-fed on organic pastures. The nutrients in eggs are healthiest when the egg white is cooked and the yolk is as runny as possible.

Beans and legumes

Beans and legumes provide protein and are a good source of fibre. The protein in beans and legumes is incomplete. If you are a vegetarian, you will need to include nuts and seeds or grains to make the protein complete. (To learn more about complete protein, see Chapter 2.) The 'In a nutshell' section below recommends the healthiest way to prepare and cook beans and legumes.

In a nutshell:

How to prepare grains, beans and legumes

If you use dried grains, beans and legumes, soak them overnight in water with the juice of half a lemon. The lemon juice helps to 'pre-digest' these foods. Pour off the soaking water before you cook these foods and add fresh water for cooking. If you have access to kombu sea vegetable add a piece to this cooking water. Kombu will help with the flatulence that eating beans can produce and adds some beneficial trace minerals. When you first bring beans to a boil, they will develop a kind of greyish scum on the top of the water. Just skim this off as it forms. Remove the kombu at this stage. If you use organic tinned beans, drain them in a colander, add a little lemon juice and after a few minutes, rinse them under running water before using them in a recipe. You do not need to pre-soak split peas or lentils for longer than an hour as they cook quickly. Soaking beans and grains overnight is beneficial for health as it removes enzyme inhibitors that occur naturally with these foods. Some people lament the fact that they forgot to soak their beans or grains the night before and now cannot have them for their dinner. There is nothing magic about night-time! The day-time equivalent to overnight is about eight hours. So if you forget to soak these foods overnight, just start soaking them in the morning and they will be ready to cook by later that afternoon.

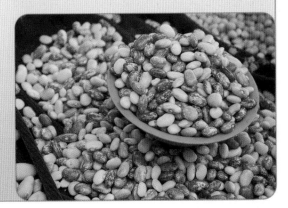

Nuts and seeds

Nuts are the seeds of trees and seeds are embryonic plants. This means that they contain within them the nutrients needed to grow a new plant. They contain protein, fats, minerals and some vitamins, such as vitamin E. Look for organic and raw nuts and seeds. Avoid the roasted and salted packaged nuts because damaged fats and poor quality salt have been added to them and the roasting has damaged their own fats. You can make nuts more digestible by soaking them overnight, draining the water and then dehydrating them in a low temperature oven. They also contain some natural enzyme inhibitors which can impede your ability to digest them. Linseeds or flaxseeds are a good source of Omega-3 fats (see Chapter 2) but you need to briefly grind them in a spice or coffee grinder before using them or they will pass through you as they have very hard shells. You can also soak them overnight and then add them to smoothies or shakes. Do not heat these seeds as their fats are easily damaged. Avoid any nuts or seeds that have mould on them. Peanuts are not nuts, they are actually legumes.

Grains

Grains are also a form of seed. Grains are mostly carbohydrate foods, but they are the complement protein to beans and legumes in a vegetarian diet. (See Chapter 2 on protein). Gluten, which is the protein found in wheat and other grains, such as barley and rye, is a common problem protein as many people find that they have a food sensitivity to it. Grains that don't have this type of gluten include rice, amaranth, buckwheat, millet, quinoa, wild rice and corn (yes, corn is actually a grain!). Kamut and spelt are older forms of wheat. Some people with wheat intolerances find that they can tolerate these grains, but they do contain gluten, so very sensitive people will not be able to tolerate them. The 'In a nutshell' section in Chapter 5 recommends the healthiest way to prepare and cook grains.

Vegetables

Incorporating a variety of vegetables in your diet is good for health. This may be the only statement about healthy nutrition that every expert agrees with! Vegetables are the parts of plants that you can eat. They are the cornerstone of a healthy diet. Vegetables are replete with vitamins, minerals, and phytonutrients, but these nutrients will be at their optimum amounts if you can eat the vegetable as close to the time it was picked as possible. If vegetables are shipped from faraway places and then stored they lose some of their nutritional value. Vegetables are also a

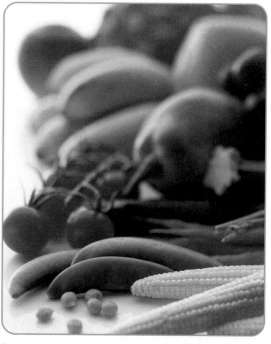

Choose a "rainbow" of coloured vegetables as part of a healthy diet

good source of fibre. Leafy green vegetables are those which have edible leaves. These include lettuce, kale, chard, spinach, and leaves of other plants such as the leaves of a broccoli. They are more delicate than other vegetables and should only be washed just before preparing and serving them. There are many more vegetables to choose from in designing your healthy diet. If you can find sea vegetables, these are a good source of minerals. The healthiest ways to prepare vegetables are to serve them raw, lightly steamed or boiled or stir-fried.

Wholefood helpers

At the beginning of this chapter we gave example of foods like apple juice and tofu that are not wholefoods but which have earned the right to be included because of their benefit to health. Like wholefoods, these foods are nutrient dense, which means that they are a concentrated source of nutrients. You might think of them as little nutrient packages. Wholefood helpers will not be a major part of your diet, but they will play a role in it. They are more like condiments, which means that they should be consumed in small amounts. These foods can be consumed sparingly and still be a part of a healthy diet.

Fats and oils

Fats and oils are wholefood helpers. You would not fill most of your plate with these foods, even if they are plant-based. But small amounts of fats and oils should be included as part of a healthy diet. The healthiest foods for cooking include butter, ghee, coconut oil and olive oil. In Chapter 2 you will learn more about the benefits of these healthy fats.

Fruits

Fruits are the part of a flowering plant that contain at least one seed. They offer vitamins, minerals, phytonutrients and fibre, but they are also high in natural sugar. Because of this, though fruit is nutritious, it should be more limited than vegetables in a healthy diet. Fresh fruit is most often eaten raw and it makes a good energising snack. It can also be cooked. Dried fruit is a more concentrated source of fruit sugar and should therefore be eaten sparingly.

Vegetable and fruit juices

Juices are a concentrated source of vitamins, minerals and phytonutrients. They should be consumed sparingly. Vegetable juices will have less of a concentration of sugar than fruit juices. Wheatgrass juice has a cleansing effect on the body but should not be taken in large amounts or it can provoke a negative reaction.

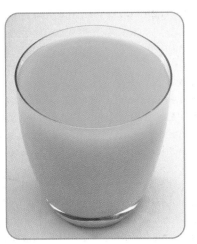

Fruit juice is good but it contains a lot of sugar

Tofu

Tofu is a protein food made from soya. In a traditional oriental diet, only small amounts of tofu are consumed at a time. For more of a discussion on soya foods, see Chapter 2.

Chocolate

Here is the statement all you chocolate lovers have been waiting to read in a book about nutrition: chocolate is good for you! Chocolate comes from cacao beans and these beans are very high in antioxidants. For chocolate to be a healthy choice, you must find some that is high in cacao with very little added sugar or fat. This will be a dark chocolate. And remember, it should only be eaten as a condiment! A reasonable amount would be not more than one/two squares a day, preferably after meals rather than as a snack.

Supplements

By now, you have probably noticed that we haven't mentioned supplementation. I am often asked if I use supplements with my clients. As a nutrition consultant, I do, but only therapeutically and for a short period of time. Some nutritionists argue that the soil our food is grown in is too depleted to offer adequate nutritive value to the foods grown in it, and I agree partly with this statement. However, I have found that by following the 'General guidelines for a healthier diet' (listed on page 5) and the more specific suggestions in the subsequent chapters, most people can maximise their ability to digest and detoxify. Organic wholefoods provide superior nutrition that is supportive in healing and in nourishing the body. No supplementation will ever take the place of wholefoods. Supplementation is just that: 'supplements' are not 'instead ofs'.

My overall recommendation regarding supplementation is to take a good quality multivitamin and mineral if you think you need it. If you feel you need additional help in the form of targeted supplementation to address a specific condition, it would be best to consult with a qualified nutritional therapist who can help you design a programme that is appropriate for you. The problem with supplementation is that interrelationships exist between nutrients. If you take one nutrient therapeutically (in high doses) it could deplete your body of another nutrient. Nutritional therapists are trained to know how to use supplementation therapeutically and will be aware of the balance that exists between specific nutrients. For suggestions on where to find a qualified nutritional therapist, see the 'Where to go from here' section, near the end of the book.

FAQs

Do I need to eat a wholefoods diet all of the time in order to be healthy?

The best way to make changes in a diet is to do so gradually. If you are currently eating a diet that mostly consists of refined processed foods it would be difficult for you to instantly change and to rigidly adopt all of the 'General guidelines for a healthy diet'. Making small changes can have a profound effect on your health and you will be more likely to incorporate these changes into your lifestyle than if you were to try to drastically change your diet all at once.

Why do we need to cook the whites of eggs but have the yolks as close to raw as possible?

The delicate nutrients found in the egg yolk are more sensitive to heat while the egg white contains substances which interfere with the absorption of a B-vitamin called biotin and which inhibit protein digestion. Cooking the egg white neutralizes these substances.

In a nutshell recipe:

Vital vegetable broth

Nutrition Notes: This broth is the cornerstone recipe for this book. It can be used as a stock for making soups and it can also be drunk as a hot or cold drink. Many people have said that they have more energy, better sleep, better skin and have experienced a soothing effect on the nervous system when they consume this broth daily.

(Use organic vegetables if possible.)
2 medium yellow onions
4 leeks (most of the green tops removed)
7 carrots
7 stalks of celery
4 red potatoes
2 sweet potatoes
12 green string beans
½ bunch of flat leaf parsley

1 bay leaf
4 cloves of garlic
12 black peppercorns
4 whole allspice
1 tablespoon sea salt

1 Wash and roughly chop the vegetables into large chunks. Do not peel – even keep the skins on the garlic and the onions.
2 Put all of the ingredients into a large pan.
3 Fill the pan with filtered water to cover the vegetables and to just a few inches below the top of the pan.
4 Cover the pan and bring to a boil. Lower the heat and simmer for at least two hours.
5 Let the mixture cool enough to handle and then strain it into containers for storing and/or a jug for drinking. To strain: use a colander lined with muslin.

Herbal therapy

As you read the rest of *Nutrition in Essence,* you will also notice that there is no mention of the use of herbs in treatment. The combination of food and herbs presents a very powerful modality for treatment and healing and I use many herbs in the form of tinctures and teas in my practice. However, it is out of respect for the practice of herbalism that I have not recommended herbs for specific conditions because I feel it would be best to consult with a qualified herbalist if you wish to incorporate herbs in a treatment.

Summary

You now have the basic general recommendations for following a healthy wholefood diet and the healthiest way to consume them. Part Two of *Nutrition In Essence* will give you more specific information about individual nutrients and how your digestion and detoxification systems work. Part Three presents specific conditions and gives recommendations for specific foods to focus on that could be helpful for these conditions. For some conditions, it may be best to avoid certain foods even if they are considered to be healthy wholefoods for most people. You will find discussions about which foods to avoid for each condition listed in Part Three of *Nutrition In Essence.*

Now let's investigate the specifics. In subsequent chapters, we will challenge some of the more widely believed dietary myths. You may want to try the suggested experiments and the wholefood recipes that are supportive of particular dietary principles. You will also find case studies about real people who successfully improved their health through a diet of wholefoods. Some of the most frequently asked questions about nutrition are presented and answered. Please read on!

nutrients in food

part two

This section of *Nutrition in Essence* introduces you to the nutrients that are found in food. All of these nutrients are essential to health. Here you will learn where to find these nutrients in foods and why they are important.

macro-nutrients

Macronutrients are the nutrients you consume in large amounts: this is the 'macro' part of the word. The three macronutrients are protein, fats and carbohydrates. These are the nutrients around which there is so much controversy concerning today's fad diets.

In this chapter you will learn about the nutritional benefits of these three macronutrients and why all three are essential for a healthy diet.

By the end of this chapter, you will be able to address the high-protein/high-fat versus high-carbohydrate/low-fat debate and you will also have read some dietary myth-busting.

Protein

Proteins in your diet are used to help all of your body grow and to repair itself when parts of it are damaged. Protein is an important component of your muscles, including your heart muscle, and your brain. Perhaps this is why the word protein comes from the Greek word '*protos*' which means 'first'. Many of your body's hormones, enzymes, parts of blood and antibodies are also proteins. Because of the many uses of proteins in the body, protein will be the first of the three macronutrients we will look at in this chapter.

The role of nitrogen

Protein is different from fats and carbohydrates because although all three macronutrients contain carbon, hydrogen and oxygen atoms, protein is the only one that contains nitrogen atoms. It is the nitrogen in protein that is the reason that high protein diets have been criticised as being unhealthy. You may wonder why this is important. (You may also be thinking that this is going to be just another chemistry lesson, but stay with it – it won't take too long.)

All life requires nitrogen and the air around us is almost 80 per cent nitrogen, but it is in a form that we cannot use. Therefore, air nitrogen must be changed into a 'fixed' form of nitrogen so that your body can use it. Nitrogen is fixed when it is combined with oxygen or hydrogen. There are two main ways in which nitrogen is fixed. One way requires certain very important bacteria. These bacteria are called nitrogen fixing bacteria. Some of them can fix nitrogen by themselves while others must first live in the roots of certain legumes before they can fix nitrogen. These bacteria fix or change the air nitrogen, then plants can take up the new form of nitrogen and make their own proteins and then animals can eat the plants and get protein from them. We can then eat plants or animals for our protein sources.

Apart from the nitrogen-fixing bacteria, there is another source in nature that fixes nitrogen – lightning! The power of lightning enables it to break the air nitrogen molecules, which then combine with oxygen molecules. These new molecules dissolve in rain and fall to the earth as nitrates. Nitrates can be taken up by plants and, again, animals eat the plants and we can eat plants or animals for our protein sources.

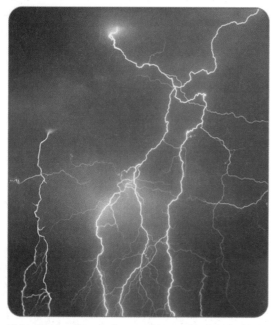

Lightning changes air nitrogren into a form that the body can use

Why we need proteins

Your body uses the protein in the foods you eat by first digesting the food and then assimilating it. For the protein part of the food you eat, your body will break it down into the small components of the protein which are known as the 'building blocks' of protein. These building blocks are called amino acids. You may enjoy eating a piece of fish for your dinner, but what your body really wants is to break down that fish and use the amino acids in the fish protein. Once your piece of fish has been digested, your body will take all of these amino acids and will line them up as building blocks and reform them into the proteins your body needs at the time. If you need to build muscle, you will build muscle. If you need to make some protein-based hormones, you will make these hormones. A child may use the amino acids from the protein they eat to support a growth spurt. A pregnant woman will use the amino acids from the protein she eats to 'build' a baby. A bodybuilder might use amino acids to build more muscle. A recently wounded person might use amino acids to make more blood.

The essential amino acids

Overall, there are about 22 amino acids, which are the building blocks of your body proteins. Eight of these amino acids are essential, which means that your body cannot make them itself and you will need to get them from your food. This is why it is so important to have some protein in your diet. If one or more of the eight essential amino acids is missing, your body will not be able to form the proteins it needs. You cannot substitute one of these building blocks for another. The other amino acids are called non-essential, because your body can make them itself by combining essential amino acids. Increasingly, there is debate among nutritionists that some of these non-essential amino acids may become essential for people who have digestive problems or who are on diets that are deficient in protein. Such people may have impaired ability to make the non-essential amino acids. (In Chapter 5 we discuss digestion and you will learn ways in which you can optimise your ability to digest your food so that you can get the nutrients you need.)

The eight essential amino acids are: isoleucine, leucine, phenylalanine, threonine, tryptophan, methionine, valine and lysine.

Animal sources of protein

Animal sources of protein are the most concentrated sources of protein and include beef, game, lamb, pork, poultry, fowl, fish and eggs.

Diet and nutrition myth: *All red meat is bad for your health*

Red meat has been singled out as a major source of heart disease and cancer. Interestingly, though the public has listened to those who have maligned red meat and consumption has dropped, the rates of these diseases have continued to climb. In many ethnic indigenous cultures red meat is consumed and rates of these diseases are low.

The dangers of red meat are most likely due to the way the animals are raised. As you read earlier, there is a big difference between factory–farmed animals that are given growth hormones and antibiotics and animals that are allowed to graze on pasture free from pesticides and fertilizers. Often, the animals raised on factory farms are given grain feed which may also have pesticides on it. These animals may also be injected with steroids and growth hormones to make them more tender and to make them grow faster. They may be given antibiotics to keep them from becoming ill due to their crowded conditions. Similar conditions are often true for poultry. The best sources of all meat and poultry are organic, free-range and pasture-fed. Fish that has been farmed and not caught in the wild may also be given antibiotics and may be fed on feed that is not organic.

The completeness of the protein you eat depends on how many of the essential amino acids there are in the food. Many nutrition experts consider eggs to be the most complete protein food, against which all others are compared. Eggs contain all eight essential amino acids. For years we have been told that we should either limit or eliminate our consumption of eggs because of their cholesterol content. However, in his book *Eat, Drink and Be Healthy*, Walter Willet, Chairman of the Department of Nutrition at the Harvard University School of Public Health, says that eggs used to be called 'the perfect food'. He also states that no research has ever shown that people who eat more eggs have more heart attacks than those who eat

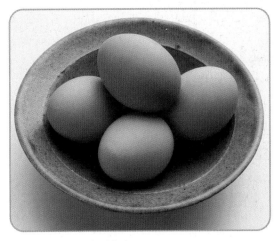

Eggs are actually healthy!

few eggs. Eggs can be very healthy sources of protein. In addition to being complete protein foods, eggs have B-vitamins, lecithin and other nutrients.

(See Chapter 10 for a discussion of the cholesterol issue.)

Dairy sources of protein

The next most concentrated sources of protein are dairy products, such as cheese, milk and yogurt. Dairy sources can include cattle, goats or sheep. The situation for dairy is the same as for meat: the healthiest sources of dairy are organic ones. If you have access to organic raw dairy, these will be the healthiest choices. Some people find they do not tolerate dairy foods well. (See Chapter 11 for a discussion on food intolerances.)

Vegetable sources of protein

Vegetable sources of protein include grains, beans, legumes, nuts and seeds. Vegetable sources of protein are not complete proteins, because they lack one or more of the essential amino acids. Therefore, if you don't eat any animal foods at all, including eggs, you need to make sure your diet contains a variety of vegetable foods so that you get the essential amino acids you need. This isn't difficult to do. For example, legumes are deficient in methionine, while grains are deficient in lysine. But grains contain methionine and legumes contain lysine. These foods contain complementary proteins, which means that you can make a complete protein by including both in your diet. You don't need to eat complementary protein foods in the same meal, but you do need to eat them within three

to four hours of each other in order to provide your body with all of the eight essential amino acids it needs.

Looking at your protein intake

Many people eat too much of the concentrated protein sources (meat, chicken, fish, eggs and dairy). Because these foods are concentrated, a serving size that is roughly the size and thickness of the palm of your hand will be enough for one meal, for most people. However, we have different needs for different amounts of protein, depending on a variety of factors, such as how old we are, how much energy we expend and what climate we are living in. Protein food is a warming food. You may need more if you are living in a colder climate than if you are in a warmer climate. In winter, you may want warming protein meals such as stews, and lighter meals in the summer. For example, an outdoor landscape gardener in Scotland, who needs muscle strength and who is living in a cold climate, might need more than the average requirement for protein.

Is it more expensive to eat organic protein?

I am often told that organic sources of meat, poultry and fish are far more expensive than non-organic sources. But you really don't have to spend much money on these foods. If you eat meat, you could choose to make just one of your meals in a day contain meat and make a stir-fry with a variety of vegetables and a piece of organic meat the size of the palm of your hand. The next day, one of your meals could contain two free-range organic eggs. This kind of meal planning would not be too costly.

When is protein in the diet a problem?

As we know, protein is a macronutrient and therefore is essential for health. However, eating too much protein can be problematic. This is really an issue of portion control and timing of eating. Overall, it is best for your body to have just the exact amounts of protein foods that it needs and to have some protein at every meal. Many people eat far more than they need, either because they are following a high-protein diet or because they have no real idea of what one portion of a protein food should be. Increasingly, when we eat out in restaurants, we are being served excessively large portions of food. This is so common a practice that many people believe that the amount of food we are served is right for one portion. If you are someone who eats meat, how often are you served a piece of meat that is only the size and thickness of the palm of your hand?

Once your body has digested the protein you have eaten and it has taken the nutrients and the amino acids that it needs from this food, the rest of the food becomes waste and your body needs to process and eliminate this waste. Here is where we will revisit our old friend nitrogen, the atom that is in protein but not in carbohydrates or fats. The waste parts of the protein food you eat will contain some nitrogen. Part of the process of eliminating protein waste involves a conversion of this nitrogen to ammonia. As you can imagine, ammonia is a highly toxic substance, so your body then converts this ammonia to a less toxic substance called urea before it is excreted through your kidneys and from your body as urine. If you eat large amounts of protein foods in excess of what you need and you do this on a regular basis, your elimination system can become overwhelmed. As the excretion of these waste products occurs through your kidneys, this is why high-protein diets are criticized as being harmful for the kidneys. The answer here is to not eat too much protein at any one meal.

Excess protein is also difficult to digest, especially if you have digestive problems (See Chapter 5). Improperly digested protein can sit in the intestines where it can putrefy and feed putrefactive (unfriendly) bacteria. Since meat has no digestive fibre, eating lots of meat can add to this problem since it will stay in the intestines longer if there is no fibre to keep it moving through. Exposure to the toxic by-products of putrefactive bacteria adds to digestive complications and can increase the risk of developing certain cancers such as colon cancer and breast cancer. You can avoid this risk by not eating too much protein at any one meal and by making sure that your general diet has enough fibre in it. Eating a wholefood diet will ensure this.

Soya as a protein source

Diet and nutrition myth: *Regular inclusion of soya in your diet provides a healthy source of protein.*

At this point, I would like to discuss soya as a protein source. This subject is controversial. Many vegetarians and vegans rely on soya as a major source of protein in their diets. Since soya has been a meat substitute for several decades, we now have scientific evidence that shows how regular use of soya in the diet affects health. For years, we have been told that soya is a healthy food because it is used in traditional oriental diets and people from these countries do not have the rates of cancer, heart disease and other degenerative disease that we do in the West. Because of this, a huge industry was born and we can now find many different food products that are soya-based. Tofu, miso and tempeh are soya foods that are traditionally eaten in countries like Japan and Indonesia, but in the West we have created soya products to resemble and replace animal foods. We now have soya milk, soya sausages, soya patties, soya cheese, and textured soya protein to use in recipes in place of minced meat. These products have been aggressively marketed to health-conscious people as low-fat, low-cholesterol protein sources which will prevent heart disease and cancer. They have also been marketed to women as foods which will help balance female hormones and prevent osteoporosis and to men as foods which will help prevent prostate cancer.

Soya and cancer

While it is true that there are lower rates of breast cancer and prostate cancer in Asian countries, if we investigate rates of diseases in these countries further, we learn that Asian countries have higher rates of cancers of the oesophagus, stomach, thyroid, pancreas and liver. If we then look at the amounts of soya that Asian countries are consuming, we see a totally different picture from the one that has been presented to us by people who are proponents of soya consumption. For example, in Japan, soya is a very small part of the Japanese diet. Along with soya, a traditional Japanese diet consists of rice and other grains, fish, vegetables, sea vegetables, fruits, nuts, pickles and other fermented foods and green tea. The historical traditional Japanese diet is primarily a wholefood diet. The more modern Japanese diet has changed to include more processed and refined foods. As in the West, cancer rates have risen in Japan

over the last fifty years, and also as in the West, the rising rates of cancer in Japan are probably due in part to the change in diet to fewer wholefoods and more processed and refined foods (though causes of cancer are seen as having many factors and certainly include environmental reasons as well).

Traditional uses of soya

Even the traditional modern Japanese diet does not contain soya in large amounts. Portions of foods are generally much smaller in Japan than in the West.

A traditional Japanese meal might consist of a small bowl of rice, a plate with some grilled fish or chicken and some grated daikon or mouli to assist with the digestion of the fat in the fish, a small bowl of miso soup with some wakame sea vegetable and a few tiny cubes of tofu, a small vegetable dish and a very small dish with a few slices of pickles to aid with digestion, and a cup of green tea. The soya contribution to this meal would be the miso soup with the small bits of tofu. Most often, miso soup is taken at breakfast and the kind of soup served with this example meal would be a broth soup with meat or vegetables. Years ago, within this meal, the rice would have been brown rice, the miso would have been made by a traditional miso-making family, the soya used in the miso would have been naturally fermented over a long period of time, and the pickles would have been naturally cultured over time as well. A naturally fermented soya food will be easier to digest. But in modern Japan, chemicals are now used to quickly ferment miso, white rice has replaced brown rice and the pickles are pickled quickly using chemicals and bright food colouring.

Soya in the West

Back in the West, soya has not only appeared in increasing amounts in foods, but concentrated

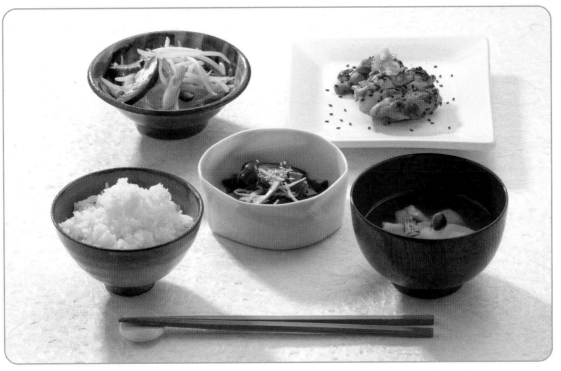

A traditional, balanced, Japanese meal

elements of soya are marketed in supplement form. You can find highly processed soya powders being sold as protein powders, and capsules of isoflavones often promoted as being hormone-balancing. You can also get soya infant formula which is promoted as being a better source for baby than a milk-based formula.

Because we now have a history of soya consumption in the West, we are seeing some of the health problems associated with it. In fact, early in 2006 a major producer of soya withdrew its petition with the US Food and Drug Administration (FDA) to be able to make cancer health claims on their food labels because the FDA advised them that they had not provided enough evidence to support the claim that soya can prevent cancer. Soya is a known goitrogen, which means that it adversely affects the thyroid gland.

Unfermented soya also contains enzyme inhibitors and phytates which block protein digestion and bind with minerals and deplete them from the body. Added to this list of ills, soya has always been on the top-ten list of foods which cause allergies.

Guidelines for eating soya

So is all the news about soya bad news for health? I don't think so. If you know that you don't have a soya allergy or sensitivity (see Chapter 11 on allergies and sensitivities) and you don't have a hypothyroid condition, then soya can be a healthy inclusion in your diet as long as you follow these guidelines:

✎ Choose soya foods that are organic and have been naturally fermented. These would include miso, tempeh, natto and soy sauce (shoyu). Preserve the integrity

21

of your fermented miso with its beneficial enzymes by not boiling it as you make it: make your soup first and add the miso after you have removed your soup from the boil.

🐝 If you eat tofu, remember that it is not a wholefood, but it is a wholefood helper, so eat it sparingly. Resist the temptation to substitute large slabs of tofu for meat in making Western dishes such as lasagne.

🐝 Avoid processed soya such as soya sausages, soya patties, soya cheese, textured vegetable protein and soya milk.

🐝 Edamame are young green soya beans which are boiled in their pods and are usually served chilled and salted. You eat them by squeezing the beans out of their pods. In Japan, they are often offered as an accompaniment to beer in beer gardens. These are wholefoods and have lower amounts of enzyme inhibitors and phytates. If you eat them, eat them as more of an accompaniment rather than in large quantity.

🐝 Avoid soya foods from oriental supermarkets which have used chemicals to ferment the food quickly. These will be cheaper than the naturally fermented foods. You will tend to find the organic, naturally fermented soya foods in health food stores.

🐝 If you are a vegetarian, include soya as only a part of your protein food consumption and include more of a variety of other protein food sources such as eggs, nuts and seeds, other beans, legumes and grains and some dairy.

casestudy: Anxious Annie

Annie was a 38-year-old client who came for a nutrition consultation because she felt that she wanted to be on a healthy diet as she got older. She wanted me to help her identify the foods that would be healthy for her to eat. In taking her case history, she told me that she was on medication for anxiety attacks. She said these attacks happened occasionally and only when she was driving, but that they were debilitating because she was finding it increasingly difficult to drive. She did not associate these attacks with her diet because they did not occur immediately after eating. However, when I asked her when in her life these attacks started, it became evident that they started at the same time she decided to include soya in her diet. Previously, she had not eaten soya but she had read in a woman's magazine that soya foods are good for balancing female hormones so she decided to give soya foods a try. Because of the association between the inclusion of soya in her diet and the onset of her anxiety attacks, I suggested that she try a trial period of three weeks without soya. Annie was amazed to discover that when she avoided soya, she did not experience anxiety attacks. She remained off soya and checked in with me from time to time after her initial experiment. Months later she still had not had a recurrence of her anxiety attacks. Her doctor took her off the medication because she no longer needed it. All she had to do was avoid soya. This is not to say that all anxiety attacks are caused by food allergies, but Annie's case is one where she had a sensitivity to soya and needed to avoid it altogether. (You will find more about food allergies and sensitivities in Chapter 11.)

Guidelines for including protein foods in your diet

Follow the 'General guidelines for a healthier diet' in Chapter 1. Also the following:

- Consider your personal needs. Do you feel that you need more protein than the suggested average portion? Or are you currently eating too much protein?

- Do not eat too much protein at one meal. Spread your protein foods throughout the day.

- Preferably choose foods that are organic and if they are animal foods, pasture-raised and free-range whenever possible.

- If you eat fish, choose fish that was caught in the wild if possible.

- If you eat eggs, choose eggs that come from organically raised, free-range poultry.

- Choose bean, legume, grain sources that are organic and prepare them as suggested in Chapters 1 and 5.

- If you eat soya, choose your soya foods based on the guidelines listed on pages 21 and 22 of this chapter.

Fats

Fats are the next macronutrient we will discuss. We will begin with another myth.

Diet and nutrition myth: *A diet which is a very low-fat or no-fat diet is a healthy diet.*

This diet myth is potentially one of the most damaging that I have ever heard health writers make. Belief in the truth of this statement has led to unnecessary suffering. Fats in the diet are essential for health. The problem with the belief that a low-fat or no-fat diet is healthy is that it does not differentiate between dietary fats. The fact is that there are healthy, necessary fats as well as the unhealthy fats, consumption of which contributes towards degenerative disease.

Consider these facts:

- About 60% of your brain is made of fat.

- The sheathes around your nerves are made of fat and fat is soothing to the nervous system.

- Fat pads out and protects your internal organs.

- Fat insulates your body and preserves your body heat.

- You need to have fat in your diet in order to be able to digest, absorb and transport vitamins A, D, E, and K in your body.

- Every cell in your body has a membrane surrounding it that is made of fat, This cell membrane is where communication between cells takes place.

Fatty acids

When we talk about fats in the diet we are really talking about fatty acids.

All fats in foods are made up of different fatty acids. If you were to write out the chemical formula for a fatty acid you would notice that they all have something in common: at one end of their chain, there is a group of three hydrogen atoms and a carbon atom, which is called a 'methyl group' in chemistry. At the other end of the chain, there is a group of two oxygen atoms, a hydrogen

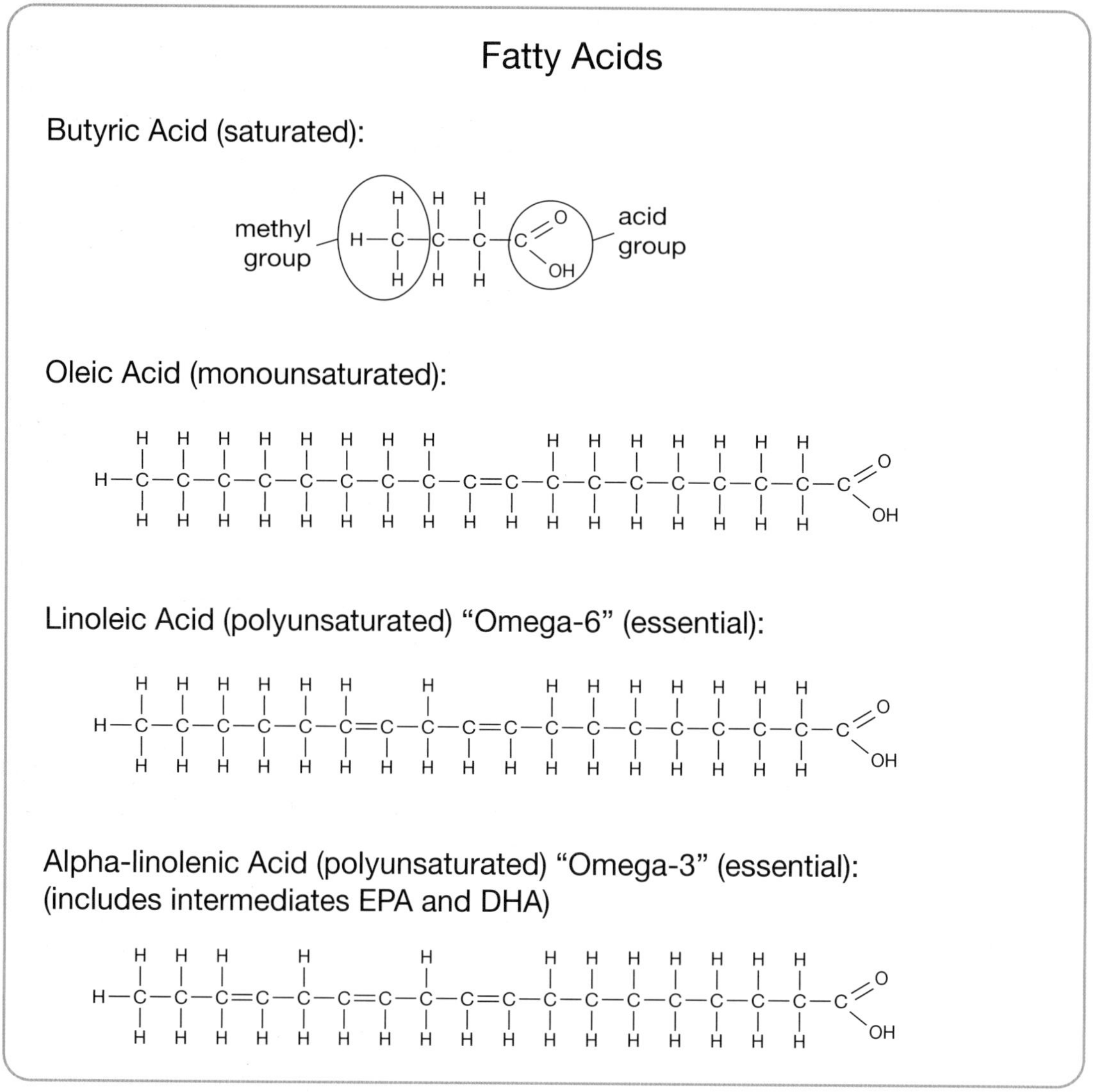

Fatty Acids

Butyric Acid (saturated):

Oleic Acid (monounsaturated):

Linoleic Acid (polyunsaturated) "Omega-6" (essential):

Alpha-linolenic Acid (polyunsaturated) "Omega-3" (essential):
(includes intermediates EPA and DHA)

Fatty acid chains

atom and a carbon atom. This is called an 'acid group'. Every fatty acid has this same structure. What is different between the fatty acids is the bit in between: the chain between these two end groups has a series of carbon atoms with hydrogen atoms above and below them. This is called the 'carbon chain'. Fatty acids have either short chains (fewer than (six carbons), medium chains (six–ten carbons) or

long chains (12–24 carbons). For example, in the figure, you will see that butyric acid is a short-chain fatty acid because it only has four carbons. Short-chain fatty acids have antimicrobial properties and are protective in this way in the intestines. Lauric acid is a medium-chain fatty acid because it contains 12 carbons. Medium-chain fatty acids are absorbed directly for energy and since they are used by the body so quickly, they do not easily contribute to weight gain. Stearic acid is a long-chain fatty acid because it has 18 carbons. Oleic acid, linolenic acid and linoleic acid are also long-chain fatty acids because they each have 18 carbons. These long-chain fatty acids are 'essential', which means that your body needs them and needs to get them from an outside source because it cannot make or form them on its own.

Other terms you will see in Figure 2.4 include 'saturated', 'monounsaturated' and 'polyunsaturated'. You have probably already heard of these terms but you might not have known what they really mean in terms of their chemical definitions. Butyric acid is an example of a saturated fatty acid. If you look closely, you will notice that every carbon atom in its chain is surrounded by a hydrogen atom (except for the acid end where there is an oxygen atom). There are no blank spaces. So the fatty acid is saturated with hydrogen atoms. Stearic acid and lauric acid are also saturated fatty acids.

However, if you look at oleic acid, you will notice that in the middle of its chain, there is an 'equal sign' and above this there are two missing hydrogen atoms. The equal sign is called a double bond. Because there is only one double bond in the oleic acid chain (the acid end does not count), oleic acid is known as a monounsaturated fatty acid because the combining form 'mono' means 'one'.

Now, if you look at linoleic acid you will see two double bonds. Alpha-linolenic acid has three double bonds. These fatty acids are known as polyunsaturated fatty acids because they have more than one double bond and the combining form 'poly' means 'many' (in these cases, 'more than one').

What does this all mean? All fats in foods contain a combination of fatty acids but they might have more of one type of fatty acid than others in their mixture. Therefore, they are often identified by the characteristics of the fatty acid that they have the most of. For example, butyric acid is the dominant fatty acid in butter. Because of this, butter is often called a 'saturated fat' even though butter also has some polyunsaturated fatty acids in it. Butyric acid is also food for the cells in your intestines, and in laboratory experiments it has actually stopped the growth of colon cancer cells! Oleic acid is the dominant fatty acid in olive oil and because of this olive oil is referred to as a monounsaturated fat. Linoleic acid is predominantly found in safflower oil so it is generally known as a 'polyunsaturated fat'. However, please remember that even though there may be a predominant fatty acid, the fats in foods are always a combination of more than one fatty acid.

Omega fats

You may heave heard of Omega-6 and Omega-3 fatty acids. These omega fats play many roles in health. Your brain, nervous system and cell membranes need these omega fats. They are also precursors to make prostaglandins: hormone-like substances in the body, some of which are anti-inflammatory.

Hard and fluid fats

A double bond makes a fat more fluid because the molecule can bend and twist at the double bond. If there is no double bond, as there is not in saturated fats, the fat is more stiff and hard. So in foods, you will notice that butter is a hard food because it is usually hard unless it is melted, while safflower oil is a liquid oil. Even if you put safflower oil in the refrigerator, it will not become hard. But what about olive oil? If olive oil is kept in a cupboard, it is an oil, but if you put it in the refrigerator it can become more solid.

Saturated fats

Diet and nutrition myth: *Saturated fats are bad for you and should be eliminated from your diet.*

When we are told that saturated fats are unhealthy fats and polyunsaturated fats are healthy fats, this is not true. We really need an array of fats in our diet. Furthermore, these kinds of statements are not taking into consideration how we store these fats and cook with them. Fats and oils do not respond well to heat, light or oxygen. Therefore, how you store and use fats and oils in cooking and eating is very important and can have a significant impact on your health. The more saturated a fat is, the more stable it is. The more polyunsaturated a fat is, the more unstable it is. Since fats will become rancid or damaged if they are exposed to heat, light or oxygen over time, the safest foods to use in cooking will be those that are more stable. Therefore, if you are going to cook with fats, using butter, ghee (clarified butter), coconut oil or olive oil are the safest. Olive oil is only one step away from being a saturated fat, so it is not quite as heat-stable as a saturated fat, but still has conferred some protection against becoming damaged when heated. No matter what fats you cook with, however, if you heat a fat or oil and it starts to smoke, throw it out – it is already damaged!

Diet and nutrition myth: *A tropical oil such as coconut oil is bad for health because it contains saturated fat and is bad for your heart.*

Coconut oil or coconut butter is a fat that has gained more popularity recently as a health-friendly oil to include in your diet. Coconut oil contains mostly lauric acid. Lauric acid is a medium-chain fatty acid because it has 12 carbons in its chain. The medium-chain

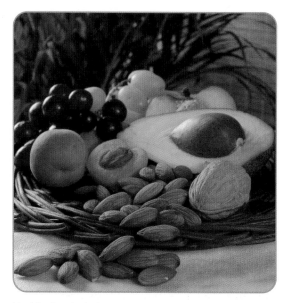

Healthy fats include coconut oil and avocado

fatty acids are burned directly for energy by the body so these fats are a direct source of energy. When you eat coconut oil, the body uses it immediately to make energy rather than store it as body fat. Sally Fallon and Mary Enig discuss the benefits of coconut oil in *Eat Fat, Lose Fat: Lose Weight And Feel Great With The Delicious, Science–Based Coconut Diet.* Lauric acid is also antifungal, antiviral and antimicrobial. It is also found in human breast milk. Coconut oil can be a useful addition to an anti-yeast diet because of its antifungal properties. Butter contains the short-chain fatty acid butyric acid which has antifungal and anti-tumour properties.

Polyunsaturated fats

If you are cooking with supermarket-bought vegetable oils, you may be using oils that are already damaged. Do your cooking oils come in clear bottles and are they stored under bright supermarket lights? Are the oils themselves clear and colourless? Natural oils are not clear and colourless.

We have been told that the polyunsaturated vegetable oils are the healthiest oils to use, but in reality these oils are easily damaged and can easily become rancid. To find the safest vegetable oils (from nuts and seeds), look for oils that say they have been expeller–expressed, are unrefined and are stored in dark glass bottles. These oils should be extracted in a process that involves low temperatures. Refined oils are extracted using high temperatures, and then they are often exposed to chemicals known as solvents. These oils may also be bleached and deodorized so that they look clean and clear and have no odour. These are damaged fats before you even open the bottle. These are the kinds of fats that can cause weight gain or heart disease.

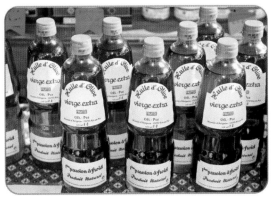
Olive oil is a healthy oil

Hydrogenated fats

The really bad fats are the fats that have been hydrogenated. Hydrogenation is a man-made process that converts a liquid oil into a hard fat. Do you remember how the saturated fats have all their carbon atom connections filled with hydrogen atoms and the polyunsaturated fats have two or more double bonds? Hydrogenation is a process whereby a liquid polyunsaturated fat such as a vegetable oil can be made into hard saturated fat by artificially filling those double-bond areas with hydrogen atoms. This is done by exposing the vegetable oils (usually cheap, already processed, damaged oils) to metal particles and then mixing this with hydrogen gas under heat and pressure. Chemicals are added to this to make this mixture have a smooth texture and then it is bleached and deodorized. Colourings and flavours are added to this to make it resemble butter in colour and taste, and *voila* – you have margarine, which is often touted as a heart-healthy health food! In reality, this process enables the food industry to use cheap vegetable oils to provide the stiffness needed in processed, baked goods, rather than using the more expensive and vastly safer butter. Hydrogenated fats created through this processing are also trans fats. This means that they have a chemical structure not known anywhere in nature.

Remember that our cell membranes are made of fat. Communication between cells happens on cell membranes. You may have read that on the surface of cell membranes are receptor sites that receive these messages from other cells and from hormones which are chemical messengers transmitting their chemical messages. Cell membranes need to have the right amount of stiffness and have the right amount of fluidity in order to function well. Saturated fats in the diet provide the stiffness and polyunsaturated fats provide the fluidity (as long as they are not rancid). Hydrogenated fats are not fats that nature understands. I believe that people who eat a diet of trans fats will have cell membranes that just don't communicate well. If you stick to a diet of wholefoods and avoid processed refined foods, you will have healthier cell membranes! Healthy cell membranes chatter easily with each other.

Flaxseeds

Flaxseeds (also known as linseeds) are good sources of Omega-3 fatty acids, but many

27

people cannot make the enzyme conversion to process them well. I still think flaxseeds are good to include in your diet if you can find them, but you would need to grind or soak them before eating them because their seed shell is so hard it would go through you without being digested if you didn't. This hard shell protects the oil inside from rancidity. I use a coffee grinder and lightly grind these seeds just before I want to use them. I sprinkle them on already cooked oatmeal and sometimes into my salads. If you drink smoothies, you can add the soaked seeds in their water to these drinks. Avoid flaxseed oil as this oil is extremely vulnerable to rancidity and even though it is sold in health food stores in a dark container and in the refrigerated section of the stores, it may still be rancid.

Guidelines for including fat in your diet

How does all this information translate into practical suggestions? Here are some general guidelines for the inclusion of the healthiest fats in your diet.

Follow the 'General guidelines for a healthier diet' and:

- Have an array of healthy fats in your diet: include some saturated, monounsaturated and polyunsaturated fats.

- For cooking, use fats sparingly and use the saturated fats. Stir fries and light sautés require little fat.

- For saturated fats, use organic butter, ghee and coconut oil if you can find it.

- Use a good quality olive oil in cooking and for salad dressings.

- As for your sources of polyunsaturated fats, remembering that these are the most vulnerable to heat, light and oxygen, don't use extracted oils, but stick to the wholefoods that contain these fats: these include raw nuts and seeds. Include raw or very lightly roasted nuts and seeds such as almonds, walnuts and pumpkin seeds in your diet.

- If you have the space, store your oils in the fridge.

- For the extremely vulnerable but essential Omega-3 fats, eat some organic wild fatty fish such as salmon, mackerel, sardines, tuna, herring, anchovies, and include pumpkin seeds, walnuts and leafy greens in your diet. Leafy greens don't have much fat in them, but they do contain a little.

- Avoid 'vegetable oil'. This is most likely rapeseed oil, also known as canola oil. Canola oil stands for 'Canadian oil'. This oil is often touted as being a healthy oil to cook with, but it is highly processed. True rapeseed has a toxic substance called erucic acid in it. Canola oil is from a rapeseed plant that has been especially bred not to have this toxic substance.

casestudy: Fat-phobic Freda

Freda was a 55-year-old woman who came for a nutrition consultation because she was in a lot of pain and wanted to know if changing her diet would help. She had severe joint pain which came on suddenly one day and was relentless. She had been to chiropractors, an acupuncturist, and several medical doctors, one of whom just gave her antidepressant medication. Nothing helped. She could not even get a proper diagnosis. In looking at her recorded diet and in questioning her, I realised that Freda was fat-phobic. Though she was slim, she lived in fear of gaining weight and was convinced that any fat in her diet would cause her to gain weight. She was very conscientious about cutting out as

much fat as she could. Her skin was also very dry. I told her all about the essential fats and that having these in her diet would be soothing to her nervous system and they would not make her gain weight. I even taught her that the essential fats are anti-inflammatory and might help with her pain and that these fats are even known to speed up metabolism and help people to lose weight. Initially, all was to no avail. Freda was not convinced and remained fat-phobic. Her pain was great, however, and she said that she had even considered suicide. Fortunately, Freda was convinced to add fats to her diet and within six weeks she was almost pain-free.

Carbohydrates

Carbohydrates represent our third macronutrient. Like proteins and fats, carbohydrates are essential. For years we were told to eat more of these than any of the other macronutrients (you may remember that they occupied the bottom tiers of the 'food pyramid'). However, there are traditional cultures, such as the Eskimos, who have managed to live on a diet that is low in carbohydrates. Like fats, carbohydrates consist of carbon, hydrogen and oxygen atoms.

Carbohydrates are your body's preferred source of energy. They consist of sugars and starches. Protein and fats can be used for energy, but if carbohydrates are present, your body will use these first. Your body breaks down all the carbohydrate in the food you eat and turns it into glucose. Glucose is a form of sugar and this becomes the fuel for all of your body's cells. You will learn more about glucose metabolism in Chapter 6.

Sources of carbohydrates

In a wholefood diet, sources of carbohydrates include grains, vegetables, fruits. There are also some in dairy products, beans and legumes. Plants have the unique ability to make their own carbohydrates through photosynthesis. The chlorophyll in their leaves allows plants to use the sun's energy to combine carbon dioxide and water to make carbohydrates.

Since carbohydrates are macronutrients for humans, you need to get them from an outside source. You do not have the ability to photosynthesise, as plants do. (Some nutritionists romantically theorise that plants were given this ability because they are rooted to the ground and cannot move around to forage for their food as humans can.) Therefore your best source of carbohydrates is plant-based foods.

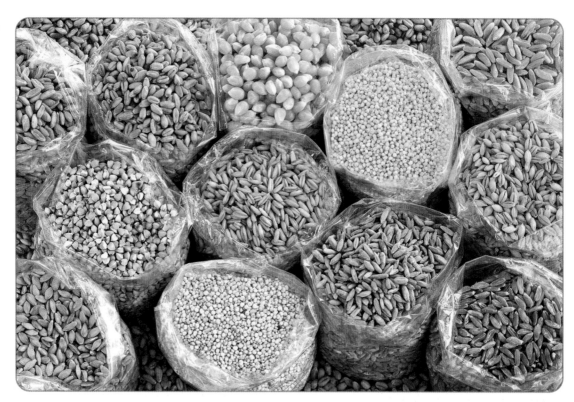

An assortment of grains

All kinds of vegetables are sources of carbohydrates. Some plants have a greater amount than others. The important thing to remember is that for good health, you should get your carbohydrates from wholefoods. Refined carbohydrates are those plant foods that have had a major part of their nutrition stripped away through processing. Eating a diet containing a lot of refined carbohydrates such as sugar and white flour not only does not add beneficial nutrients to your body, it can actually strip stored nutrients that you already had, in order to digest and metabolise them.

When you are choosing your carbohydrate foods for health, remember the definition of wholefoods. Some food manufacturers advertise their products as being wholegrain, but this does not necessarily mean they are wholefoods. For example, if you eat a type of

boxed, flaked grain cereal for breakfast, you might think you are making a healthy choice if it says it is a 'wholegrain'. But as you have already learned, this is a processed food. These grains have been heated and cooked under pressure. This makes them more difficult to digest. It is better to eat a wholegrain that is also a wholefood, such as a bowl of brown rice, or a bowl of non-instant oatmeal.

In Chapter 6 you will learn more about how carbohydrates metabolise in the body. You may want to know which vegetables are low-carbohydrate vegetables and which are high-carbohydrate vegetables. A general rule is that the root vegetables are the higher-carbohydrate vegetables. Eating these vegetables can be very helpful if you want to give up eating refined sugar, because these vegetables are sweet.

High-Carbohydrate Vegetables	Low-Carbohydrate Vegetables
Squashes	Bean sprouts (alfalfa, mung etc.)
Yams	Cucumber
Potatoes / sweet potatoes	Asparagus
Parsnips	Leafy greens (kale, spinach, chard, lettuces)
Pumpkins	Cabbage / Cauliflower / Broccoli
Turnips	Tomatoes
Beets	Artichoke / Jerusalem artichoke
Corn	Bell peppers / Hot peppers / Chillies
Peas	Mushrooms
Carrots	Aubergine
Swedes	Radishes
	Celery
	Onions / Leeks / Spring onions/Garlic
	Green beans / Snow peas
	Brussels sprouts
	Herbs (Parsley, Dill, Chives etc.)

In a nutshell recipe:

Garden green soup

This recipe gives you a chance to incorporate the Vital Vegetable Broth recipe from Chapter 1 into a soup recipe. This recipe contains a powerhouse of nutrients from vegetables. With this blended, velvety soup, even those who hate vegetables will be purring as they sip it! This soup is also very good served chilled.

2 tbsp extra virgin olive oil
55g spring onions – the white parts and some of the green parts, finely chopped
600g of English cucumber, peeled and roughly chopped
150g potato, peeled and diced
1 tsp sea salt
$1\frac{1}{2}$ pints of Vital Vegetable Broth
$\frac{1}{2}$ tsp dried dill weed
100g of young, fresh spinach leaves
Juice of half a lemon

1 tsp maple syrup
175 ml half and half cream

1 Heat the oil in a soup pan. Add the spring onions and sauté until the onions have wilted.
2 Add the cucumber, potato and the sea salt. Sauté for 5 minutes.
3 Add the vegetable broth and the dill weed.
4 Simmer until the cucumber and the potato are tender.
5 Add the spinach. Simmer until the spinach has cooked but still retains its dark green colour.
6 Add the lemon juice and the maple syrup.
7 Blend the soup in a blender until smooth. (Safety tip: fill the blender no more than three-quarters full with hot liquid and be sure the top is tightly fitted.)
8 Pour the blended soup back into the pan and stir in the cream.
9 Season to taste with more sea salt and maple syrup if needed.

Guidelines for including carbohydrate foods in your diet

Here are some guidelines about how to include the healthiest carbohydrate foods in your diet:

- Choose wholegrains, beans and legumes that are also wholefoods rather than processed. Follow the directions for preparing them in Chapters 1 and 5. The exceptions are split peas and lentils, which do not need to be soaked for as long.

- Include some leafy greens (cooked or raw) in your diet every day.

- Eat a diet that includes vegetables of different colours. This will give you a full array of all the nutrients that vegetables have to offer.

- If you can find them, include some naturally cultured vegetables in your diet (e.g. unpasteurised organic sauerkraut).

- Choose whole fruits, rather than fruit juice.

- If you have access to them and you enjoy them, include some sea vegetables (such as kombu and wakame) in your diet. They are a wonderful source of minerals.

FAQs

I love omelettes, but if I want to follow the advice of eating eggs with runny yolks and cooked whites, how can I eat them? What are the best cooking methods for cooking eggs?

Remember, these are only guidelines. They are meant to inform you as to the best methods of eating and preparing foods in order to maximise the nutrient value of these foods. The best cooking methods for cooking and preparing eggs are to boil or poach them. If you wish to follow these guidelines and you want a super-healthy omelette, here's what you can do. Lightly sauté some vegetables such as spinach, tomatoes, onions and mushrooms in a little healthy fat such as butter, olive oil, coconut oil or ghee. Separate the eggs and beat the whites and the yolks. Add the whites to the vegetables. Cook them until they are just cooked and then add in the yolks. Add seasoning and cook the yolks only for a minute or so. Fold over the omelette and enjoy.

From reading your recommendations, I am wondering if the traditional but much maligned 'English fry-up' might be actually a healthy breakfast choice?

It can be. Choose organic ingredients. Lightly fry the eggs in a healthy fat (as described above) until the whites are cooked but the yolks are still runny. Broil some tomatoes and lightly sauté some mushrooms. You can also bake some organic free-range sausages. You could even add in some puréed spinach and include a cup of hot Vital Vegetable Broth to have a healthy breakfast.

I've been to a farmer's market and bought a lot of vegetables. What is the best way to store them?

You can wash or brush the dirt off the root or tuber vegetables, such as carrots and potatoes, dry them well and store them in a cupboard or basket, with air circulating. Don't leave potatoes in plastic bags, or they will sprout and go mouldy. Leafy greens are more delicate and should not be washed until you are ready to use them. Put them in plastic bags, add just a drop or two of water, seal and label the bags and snip the bags in several places to make 'breathing holes'. Store them in the refrigerator.

I hate to admit this but I really don't like vegetables. I know they are good for me. How can I start to bring them into my food plan?

Drinking your vegetables might be a good first step towards incorporating them into your diet. Why not start by making the Vital Vegetable Broth recipe? Try drinking it as a hot drink, or as a cold substitute for some of your water quota. Once you feel a little more adventurous, use this broth as the stock for a blended soup. You might also try the roasted root vegetable recipe found in Chapter 6. Many former vegetable-haters like this recipe because roasting makes the vegetables sweet.

micro-nutrients

In this chapter we will discuss micronutrients. Micronutrients are vital for health but we need them in very small amounts: milligrams or micrograms rather than grams. These micronutrients are our vitamins and minerals.

Some nutrition books give a general listing of each and every vitamin and mineral and suggest amounts that we need every day. We take a different approach here, because we are advocating health-promoting wholefoods which contain an array of these nutrients in the ratios that are found in nature. Because we are addressing the micronutrients that are available through food, and as this is a general discussion about these nutrients, not all nutrients are discussed here.

Supplements

This book recommends getting the nutrition you need from food. If you have special conditions that could be addressed through the use of supplementation, it is suggested that you consult a nutritional therapist for your specific supplement needs.

What vitamins and minerals do

Vitamins and minerals are nutrients that act as coenzymes or cofactors in important metabolic activities that occur in your body. As a coenzyme, a vitamin helps an enzyme to work. Enzymes are special proteins that change the rate of chemical reactions in your body. Enzymes are their own energy source, which means that they don't need an outside source of energy to work and they don't need to change their forms while they are working.

There are hundreds of enzymes in your body, but the ones you might be most familiar with are your digestive enzymes. You need your digestive enzymes to be able to metabolise or break down the food you eat. Enzymes are very specific and each enzyme works only on one substance. For example, the digestive enzyme lipase only works on metabolising fat: it will not help with metabolising carbohydrates or protein. Some enzymes need to have specific vitamins present in order to do their work. These vitamins and minerals are coenzymes to their enzyme partners. If a vitamin or mineral acts as a cofactor, that means that the vitamin or mineral, plus another substance, create a specific reaction in some body process.

Vitamins

Vitamins are necessary for many of your body processes to work properly. You can develop nutritional deficiencies if you don't get the amounts that you need. A well-known vitamin deficiency disease is scurvy, which is caused by a deficiency of vitamin C. In 1795, the British Navy began giving lime juice to its sailors on long sea voyages to prevent scurvy. (This is also why these sailors were called 'limeys'.)

A named deficiency disease is the most severe form of a deficiency of a particular vitamin. However, we know today that even if you don't have a disease as severe as scurvy, you might have a nutrient deficiency to a lesser degree, due to a poor diet, demands on your body that deplete nutrients or perhaps lifestyle choices such as smoking or drinking alcohol, which deplete the body of nutrients. Some nutrition books advocate taking a variety of supplements to make up for any possible deficiencies. Beyond a general multivitamin/ mineral supplement, if you want to know if you need any specific nutritional therapy, it would be best to seek the advice of a nutritional therapist. The important thing to

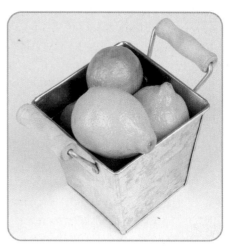

Lemons and limes contain vitamin C

remember, though, is that you cannot live on nutritional supplements alone. You need food, not only to provide you with nutrients like vitamins, but also to help your body to use these nutrients. For example, you need some dietary fat to be able to transport the fat-soluble vitamins in your body. Though supplements can be useful tools in nutritional therapy, they cannot take the place of food.

The fat-soluble vitamins

The fat-soluble vitamins are vitamins A, D, E and K. 'Fat-soluble' means that they are found in the fat component of vegetable and animal sources of foods. Fat-soluble vitamins can be stored in your body tissues and therefore it is possible to take in toxic excessive amounts of these vitamins as supplements, but not generally through food.

Vitamin A

Retinol is the form of vitamin A that originates from animal sources. Beta-carotene is the

vegetarian source of vitamin A and it is converted to retinol in the body. The absorption and conversion of beta-carotene is not as efficient as that of retinol. The main functions of vitamin A are to promote vision, including night vision, but vitamin A is also an antioxidant; it is good for skin and it supports reproduction and growth. It is also good for the respiratory system. The best food sources for vitamin A and beta-carotene are: liver, fish liver oils, eggs (the yolks) and dairy foods. Dark leafy greens or orange and yellow vegetables such as spinach, kale, chard, pumpkin, butternut squash, sweet potato and carrots are good sources of beta-carotene. Too much beta-carotene in the diet can turn your skin an orange colour. This is harmless but is an indication that you are not converting all of the beta-carotene into vitamin A. This usually only happens if you are consuming a lot of concentrated beta-carotene, such as when drinking large amounts of carrot juice.

Vitamin D

Vitamin D is technically a hormone as it is formed in one place in the body but carries out its action in another. This vitamin can be synthesized by the body through exposure of the skin to sunlight. Its main functions are to assist in bone growth through the regulation of calcium metabolism. The best source of vitamin D is exposure to sunlight, but because of fears about skin cancer and the heavy use of sunblock lotions, some cases of vitamin D deficiency have been reported. You do not need to be exposed to the sun for very long for your body to make vitamin D. Food sources of this vitamin include oily fish, fish liver oil such as cod liver oil, butter, egg yolks, liver and other organ meats.

Vitamin E

This vitamin is another antioxidant vitamin. It helps to protect your cell membranes, which are made of fat. It also protects other fats and oils from oxidizing and becoming rancid, so you could squeeze one capsule of vitamin E into your olive oil bottle to help preserve it. Your best food sources of vitamin E are cold–pressed oils, nuts, sunflower seeds, avocado, sweet potatoes, dried beans, butter, milk fat, liver and egg yolk. Vitamin E has some anti–blood-clotting properties which can be very beneficial. However, it is not advised that you take this vitamin as a

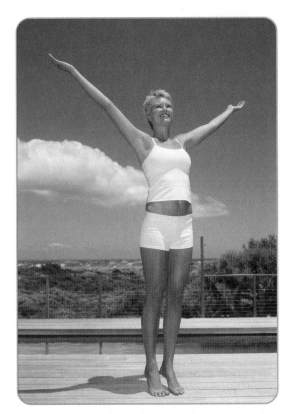

The sun helps you to make vitamin D

supplement if you are on blood thinning drugs or for a week before or after surgery.

Vitamin K

Good bacteria in your intestines can make this vitamin for you. The main function of vitamin K is to assist with blood-clotting. The best food sources of vitamin K are leafy green vegetables, liver, milk, egg yolks and fish oil. Factors that help you to maintain healthy intestinal flora will help you to make more vitamin K as well (see Chapter 5). It is thought that newborn babies might be at risk of bleeding because when they are born their intestines are sterile until they begin to grow their good flora. This is another reason to promote breastfeeding: mother's milk encourages the growth of healthy intestinal flora.

The water-soluble vitamins

The water-soluble vitamins are not stored by the body and therefore excess of these vitamins is generally washed from your body through your urine.

B-complex vitamins

Even though the B-complex vitamins have specific individual functions, they are considered as a group because they work best as a group. The individual B vitamins are B1 (thiamin), B2 (riboflavin), B3 (niacin), B5 (pantothenic acid), B6 (pyridoxine), B12 (cobalamin), folate, and biotin. The B vitamins facilitate the work of every cell. They are greatly involved in energy production in the body and needed to metabolise carbohydrates, fats and proteins. The best food sources for B-complex vitamins in general are wholegrains, vegetables, fresh fruits, nuts, legumes and seafood. Folate is important during pregnancy – deficiency can result in neural tube defects in babies, such as spina bifida. This is one supplement that your doctor might recommend if you are pregnant. B-complex vitamins are separated from grains when the grains are refined. So eating refined foods and sugar actually depletes your body of B vitamins as your body is called upon to use any reserves it has to digest and metabolise these foods.

Highlighting Vitamin B12

Vitamin B12 is found in animal foods. There is some controversy about whether or not it is also found in plant foods. The controversy lies in the argument surrounding whether B12 can be found in fermented plant foods, such as miso and tempeh. Some nutritionists argue that the source is the bacteria found in the traditional production processes and that with the introduction of modern sanitary methods, most of the beneficial bacteria has disappeared from these plant foods. Vegetarians, who eat some animal products, such as eggs, will be getting B12 in their diet. Vegans (who eat no animal products) need to ensure they have a reliable source. I have had clients who have been found to be deficient in this very important vitamin. Your body can store Vitamin B12 for a number of years, but if you do not have a reliable source or cannot absorb it well, you may become deficient. People who are deficient in this vitamin often must receive regular injections of it. If you don't eat any animal products you might want to consider taking a supplement of this vitamin.

Another cause of vitamin B12 deficiency is low production of stomach acid. Stomach acid is necessary to produce a substance that helps your body to absorb vitamin B12. (Chapter 5 looks at the importance of maximising your digestion.)

Vitamin C

This vitamin is also an antioxidant. It is known as the antiviral vitamin. Most animals on the planet (except humans and a few others) can make their own vitamin C and do so especially when they are exposed to viruses. Vitamin C protects iron from oxidation, protects your tissues, is involved in collagen synthesis, strengthens your resistance to infection and helps to combat the negative effects of stress. Good food sources of vitamin C include citrus fruits, cantaloupe, strawberries, papayas, mangoes, leafy green vegetables, broccoli, tomatoes and peppers. Vitamin C is better absorbed if there are substances called bioflavonoids with it. Interestingly, bioflavonoids are also found in these foods but mostly in the pulp and not in the juice, illustrating that it is better to get your vitamin C from wholefood sources.

Minerals

Minerals are the substances that come from the earth. They cannot be destroyed through cooking. They perform many functions in the body. in this chapter, we will consider some minerals In partnerships because they exist this way in the body. This is one reason why it is important not to overdose yourself on supplements that have high therapeutic amounts of single nutrients. You can deplete yourself in a partner nutrient if you do this over a long period of time.

Let's look at our first mineral partners.

Sodium and potassium

Both of these minerals are involved in water-balance regulation in the body. There is a theory that we came to favour potassium in our cells when we evolved to where cells first had membranes, differentiating their inside and outside environments. Fluid inside the cell

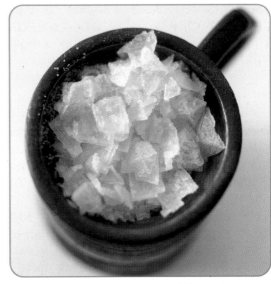

Sea salt is a good source of sodium

prefers a higher concentration of potassium, while fluid outside the cell prefers a higher concentration of sodium.

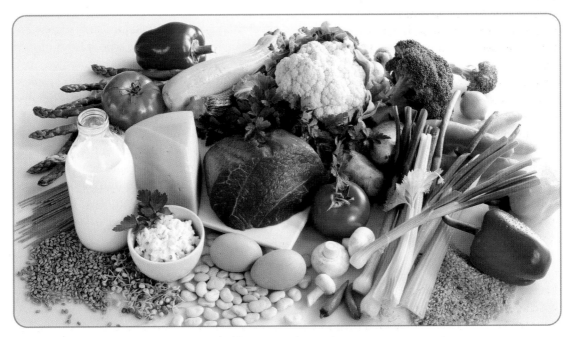

Dark green vegetables, milk and meat are valuable sources of potassium

They are also involved in nerve transmission and muscle contraction. Potassium is found in high amounts in most vegetables. It isn't usually a problem to find sodium in any diet. The most important consideration for sodium is the source. There is a world of difference between refined 'table' salt and a good quality, unrefined sea salt.

Regular inclusion of the Vital Vegetable Broth in your diet will add to your daily intake of potassium and other beneficial minerals.

Calcium and magnesium

These minerals are both involved in maintaining bone structure. Bone cells are continually broken down and rebuilt. Calcium forms the hardness on the collagen matrix when bone is made. Calcium and magnesium are also involved in muscle contraction, the transmission of nerve impulses and blood pressure maintenance. Magnesium is involved in bone mineralization and in over 300 of the body's enzyme systems, including the enzyme that allows calcium into the cell. These minerals maintain a balance with each other. Good food sources of these minerals include nuts and seeds, legumes, dark green vegetables, seafood, sea vegetables, meat, poultry (especially the dark meat) and sea salt. Chocolate cravings can be a sign of magnesium deficiency! Magnesium is known as the 'relaxer' because it relaxes muscles. Calcium levels in the body are all about absorption and deposition, not about the amounts taken by mouth.

Zinc

Zinc is important in enzyme function as it is a cofactor involved in even more enzymes than magnesium. It is often a depleted mineral due to the way foods are grown (in zinc-deficient soil). Zinc is an important cofactor for many enzymes, and it is also an important mineral for mental development, reproductive organ health (high amounts of zinc are found in healthy sperm), blood sugar control, and it helps protect the body from the toxicity of heavy metal exposure (mercury, lead, cadmium). Zinc is also important in thyroid function, the immune system and wound healing. Good food sources of zinc include oysters, red meat, nuts, seeds, fish, wholegrains and sea salt. Since zinc is a very important mineral needed for the reproductive system, perhaps this is why oysters have the reputation for being an aphrodisiac as they are quite high in zinc! Another interesting association with zinc is its connection to taste: people who are deficient in zinc often find that their sense of taste is diminished. Since refined foods are stripped of minerals like zinc, people who have a history of eating these foods and then switch to a wholefood diet sometimes initially complain of the blandness of these foods. That is because refined processed foods often have had lots of sugar and salt added to enhance their taste. But after someone has been on a wholefood diet that is naturally rich with minerals including zinc, their taste buds wake up and they find that these foods truly are delicious!

Iodine

The presence of iodine in the body is very important for two main thyroid hormones and therefore iodine is important for metabolism and the rate at which energy is released. It is also involved in making sex hormones and in fat metabolism. Good food sources of iodine include sea vegetables, sea salt, seafood, dairy and plants and animals grown or raised on iodine-rich soil. Iodized salt (store-bought salt) can actually hinder the thyroid. Goitre is an enlargement of the neck that occurs in iodine deficiency due to a thyroid enlargement. Goitrogens are foods that can depress the action of the thyroid: these foods include cabbage, cauliflower, broccoli, kohlrabi, Brussels sprouts or soya. This is really only a problem if these foods are consumed in great amounts and for someone who has a problem with low thyroid.

Selenium

Selenium is an antioxidant mineral. It acts with vitamin E to protect the immune system. It is protective against heart disease which is associated with exposure to free radicals and oxidation. (You can learn more about free radicals and oxidation in Chapter 12.) Selenium works with an enzyme to prevent free radical formation. Good food sources of selenium include Brazil nuts, seafood, meat and grains that have been grown in selenium-rich soil.

We know of the power of selenium through studies done in China, in an area where a certain type of heart disease was rampant. The soil in that part of China was depleted of selenium. At the time of writing, research has begun involving a possible connection between avian flu and the low selenium levels in the soil of China.

Chromium

Chromium is best known for its role in regulating blood-sugar levels. It helps to facilitate glucose (sugar) uptake into cells for energy and enhances the action of insulin. Good food sources of chromium include brewer's yeast, liver, nuts, wholegrains, meats and cheeses. Chromium is a part of 'Glucose Tolerance Factor' (GTF) which is a tri-part molecule that enhances glucose uptake into cells for energy. (NB: Nutritional chromium is totally different to the type featured in a film where industrial chromium is responsible for poisoning a town of people.)

Iron

Iron is important in the treatment of anaemia (iron-poor blood). Anaemia is a serious condition. But it is also important not to supplement yourself with too much iron just because you think it is healthy. Iron oxidizes easily in the body and this creates free radicals. Good food sources of iron include eggs, fish, liver, meat, sea vegetables and green leafy vegetables. These food sources include the antioxidants necessary to neutralize free radicals.

This is a brief survey of some of the key micronutrients that are essential for your health. It is important to remember that a varied wholefood diet will provide you with an array of these micronutrients, in the ratios in which nature provides them.

FAQ

I am an older woman worried about osteoporosis. Should I take calcium supplements?

For answers regarding supplementation for specific conditions, you need to seek the advice of a nutritional therapist, who will be able to evaluate your dietary history. Calcium metabolism is a complex issue and ensuring an appropriate intake involves more than just taking calcium supplements. There are cultures in the world whose intake of dietary calcium is lower than that of Western cultures, yet they have little evidence of osteoporosis. One factor that people in these cultures have in common is that they consume more wholefoods than Westerners do, and their diets do not contain nutrient-robbing refined foods.

special nutrients

You won't find a chapter about special nutrients in most books about nutrition. But we feel that these nutrients are as important as the macronutrients and the micronutrients. Let's begin this chapter by investigating another 'diet and nutrition myth'.

Water

Diet and nutrition myth: *You should drink two litres of water every day.*

This another diet myth that most of us have seen. However, when researchers decided to investigate where this specific amount came from they could not find a scientific source.

We do know that water is very important for the body. It is estimated that our bodies are between 60 and 70 per cent water. We lose water through sweat, urine and through the process of breathing, and we need to replenish it. All of our bodily fluids, including blood, urine, sweat, tears and the fluids within and between all of the cells, are primarily made of water. Water is necessary for good digestion, keeps skin and mucous

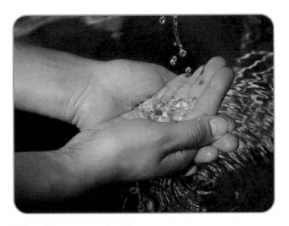

Water is necessary for life

membranes moist and helps us to get rid of toxins.

If you don't have the water you need, you may experience some of the symptoms of dehydration. These symptoms can include thirst, headache, joint or muscle pain, dry skin, backache and constipation (though there can be other medical reasons for these symptoms as well as dehydration). If you are dehydrated you might also notice that your urine is a darker yellow in colour and it might even have a strong odour. (Another reason for having dark urine is if you are taking a vitamin supplement that contains riboflavin. Vitamin B2 tends to make urine a bright yellow colour).

So how much should I drink?

How much water you should drink depends on your level of activity, the kinds of activities you undertake, the climate you are living in and the type of foods and drinks you consume. For example, if you are an athlete, you will need to drink more water than a person who is sedentary because you will sweat more and will therefore lose water more quickly. The same would apply if you like to take regular saunas at your gym or health club. If you are living in the tropics, or you go on holiday to a hot country, your need for an increase in your water consumption will be greater. Similarly, you might live in a temperate country but the indoor heating in the winter makes you feel drier than at those times of year when the heat is off. If you eat a lot of dehydrated foods such as 'trail mixes', biscuits, nuts or dried fruits, your need to drink water might be greater than if you tend to eat more watery foods, such as

salads with a lot of lettuce, celery, cabbage, spinach; or watery fruits, such as watermelon and strawberries. So, if you are an athlete, live in the tropics, take saunas on a regular basis and eat a lot of biscuits then you will need to drink a lot of water!

Certain substances can have a dehydrating effect on the body by causing the body to produce more urine and therefore to excrete more water. These substances include caffeine and some herbs and medications which are diuretics. Alcohol is also very dehydrating for the body.

People who follow special diets, such as a macrobiotic diet, believe that if you are living in a temperate or cooler climate, you do not need to drink water at all because you can get enough from the soups and salads you eat. They even believe that drinking excess water may cool the body down too much and might make you tend to catch colds more easily.

However, it has been my experience that most of my clients are dehydrated to some degree. I believe that this is because many of my clients engage in some of those dehydrating activities mentioned above and they tend to consume dehydrating substances. When I look at my clients' dietary intake records, I often notice that they are not drinking water even when they think they are. This is because they count all the fluids they consume as meeting some of their daily need for water. Again, watery foods, soups and stews can be counted as part of your daily water intake, but you need to weigh these against any dehydrating substances you might consume: that pint at the pub after work does not count as part of your daily intake of water!

What kind of water is best?

I am often asked what kind of water is the best water to drink. These days I usually advise against drinking water straight from the tap. Tap water has been treated to keep the population safe from harmful bacteria or germs. While this is a good thing, the chemicals used to kill these germs are not beneficial for health. Chlorine is the most well known of these chemicals. If chlorine is consumed on a regular basis, it can deplete the body of certain vitamins and it can also harm the beneficial flora that we have in our intestines. Though chlorine is a powerful chemical agent used to kill bacteria, it does not distinguish between the 'good bacteria' that we want and the 'bad bacteria' that can cause disease.

Filtered water

You can use tap water and remove most of the chlorine and other chemicals in it by purchasing a jug that has a built-in filter. You fill the jug with water from your tap and as the water fills the jug, it passes through the filter. These jugs are not very expensive, but you do need to change the filter on a regular basis. If you want a more powerful filter, there are more expensive filtration systems which can be installed under your kitchen sink. These systems are usually combination filtration systems, consisting of a charcoal filter and a reverse–osmosis filter. These systems can be pricey, but they do a very good job of removing almost everything from your tap water. The filters in these systems also need to be replaced from time to time. Some people believe that boiling water will get rid of any harmful chemicals. Boiling water is a useful practice for killing harmful germs but it does not necessarily get rid of harmful chemicals. In fact, boiling water can even concentrate these chemicals.

Well water

Well water can be a good source of drinking water because it has beneficial minerals in it. However, there is also the possibility of contamination from agricultural run-off and if the well water has not been treated for harmful germs. If you have a well, you might want to get the water tested. If it is free from germs and pollutants, well water is a healthy drinking water option.

Hard water

Some areas of the country have hard water. Hard water is water that naturally has a lot of minerals in it. While this can be beneficial for health, many people don't like hard water because it leaves a mineral residue in their pipes and it does not allow shampoos and soaps to lather well. These people may install a water softener in their homes. Most water softeners work by exchanging sodium for the other minerals in the water. This will allow your shampoo to make more suds, but it is not good drinking water because it will be high in sodium.

Distilled water

Distilled water is water which has been heated until it is steam and then the steam is collected and condensed. Distilled water is essentially pure water. While drinking distilled water may seem like a good idea, it isn't. Because distilled water is devoid of any minerals, it tends to attract and pull minerals from the body.

Cooking foods in distilled water pulls the minerals out of the foods and makes them less nutritious. Drinking distilled water on a regular basis could result in a loss of important minerals from your body.

Spring water

Spring water is water that comes from natural springs in the earth. Water companies collect this water, disinfect it and bottle it. Similarly, mineral water is sold as bottled water. Most natural water contains minerals, so in one sense these waters are all mineral waters. There is an increasing number of companies who are in the business to collect, bottle and sell water. They usually advertise their source as being from a special, pristine water source. They may be good sources of drinking water. The quality depends on the source, how the water has been treated and handled and whether the company has added anything to it. It is best to read the labels on these bottles to see what they contain, other than water. These days, experts are beginning to question whether storing water in soft plastic bottles is a good idea. Some believe that chemicals in the plastic may leech out into the water.

Guidelines about water

By now, you may be confused by all the options available as drinking water and you may still be wondering if you need to increase your daily intake of water. Here is a summary of the recommendations:

- Don't drink water directly from the tap: get an inexpensive jug with built-in filter and keep it filled and in your fridge. Don't forget to change the filter as the manufacturer suggests.
- You can also drink bottled water from a reputable company.
- If you have a well and want to drink your well water, get it tested first.
- Don't drink or cook food in distilled water.
- If you have a water softener in your home, don't drink this water. Find another source for drinking or get a filter for the water you drink.

As you can see from the following case study, *how* you drink water is just as important as how much or the kind of water you drink.

casestudy: Joan the water-gulper

Joan (41), was a client who I felt could benefit from adding more water to her diet. She was fairly active, worked out in a gym several days a week and had a stressful office job. Her diet intake record showed no evidence that she drank water and she complained of dry skin and tiredness. Joan told me that she hated drinking water as it was too bland. Nonetheless, she said she would try a two-week experiment in increasing her daily water intake. Only three days had gone by before I received a phone call from Joan, who was very annoyed with me. She said: 'I am trying your water experiment and I find that I have to pee all the time. I don't have the time for this! Furthermore, all this water makes me feel sick to my stomach.' As I had only asked her to increase her water intake from virtually nothing to two litres in total per day (including the amount of liquid foods she consumed, such as soups), I could not understand why she would react in this way. Finally, it dawned on me to ask: 'How and when are you drinking your water?' Joan told me that since she hated water, she wanted to get the daily drinking of it over with, so when she got up in the morning, she went to the kitchen and drank almost her full day's quota right then and there! This much water at once was too much for her body to handle – it took what it needed and excreted all the rest through her urine. This manner of drinking was an assault to her system and made her feel ill. I hadn't spelled out that she should sip her water throughout the day. That way, her body could use it better, she would not have to pee as much and it would be unlikely that she would feel nauseous.

I suggested that Joan buy a sports water-bottle with a lid and a straw and that she measure how many refills it would take for her to drink two litres of water in a day. She had a bottle that held a third of a litre, so she should aim to fill her bottle six times to meet her daily goal. I then told her to put six rubber bands around her bottle. Each time she drank the water in her filled bottle, she could remove one of the bands. That way, she would know when she had reached her quota for the day. Joan found that when she carried her bottle of water with her, and drank throughout the day, it was much more bearable. She enjoyed the feeling of success whenever she got to remove one of the rubber bands. Of course, they all had to be put back on the bottle the next day! Over time, Joan began to feel the benefits of drinking more water. She also discovered that water was not such a bad drink.

Making water more enjoyable:

- Try having a glass of room-temperature water with the juice of half a lemon squeezed into it by your bedside at night. When you wake up in the morning, sip this slowly. It is refreshing and can be a nice way to help your body greet the day.

- To your jug of filtered water in your fridge, add some lemon and lime slices or some cucumber which has been sliced lengthwise. This flavouring can help to make water more palatable.

- Try letting your body be your guide in determining how much water you should drink every day rather than believing in a magic amount.

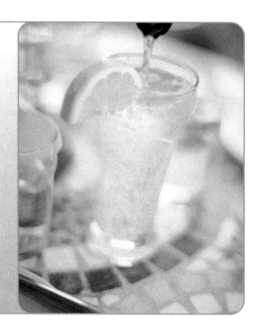

Fibre

Fibre is not a nutrient, but it is very important to have enough of it in your diet. It is estimated that our primitive ancestors ate far more fibre in their diets than we do today. They ate the wholefoods that they found in nature. These foods naturally contain good amounts of fibre. A modern diet tends to contain more refined foods and therefore we may not have much fibre in our diets.

If fibre is not a nutrient, what is it and why is it important for you to have in your diet? Fibre is the part of the plant food that you eat that your body cannot digest. At first glance, this implies that fibre is just a waste product of your food and therefore not necessary. However, fibre plays an essential role in health.

Dr. Denis Burkitt was a British surgeon who worked in Africa in the 1950s. He noticed that Africans who ate their traditional wholefoods diet did not tend to suffer from diseases of the digestive system such as constipation, haemorrhoids, diverticulitis and IBS (irritable bowel syndrome), nor did they have high rates of diabetes or heart disease. However, if these same Africans ate a modern Western diet, they developed these diseases to the same extent that we in the West have them. From his research studies, Dr. Burkitt concluded that the reason Africans who ate their traditional diet did not develop these diseases was because of the higher levels of fibre in their diets.

Soluble and insoluble fibre

The fibre found in plant foods comes in two forms: insoluble and soluble. Insoluble fibre is what we also call 'roughage', though it does have the ability to absorb some water and therefore it gives stools more bulk and makes them softer. Insoluble fibre is a bit like a broom that sweeps through your large intestine, keeping it clean and free from a build-up of toxins. In this way, insoluble fibre also decreases the time that stools remain in the large intestine and keeps things moving! This movement of food through the large intestine is one of the reasons fibre helps avoid constipation. Soluble fibre is more dissolvable in fluid and helps you to maintain more stable blood-sugar levels, lower your cholesterol levels, feel fuller after eating; and, like insoluble fibre, it reduces your exposure to toxins.

Foods that contain fibre

Both insoluble fibre and soluble fibre are found naturally in wholefoods. Foods especially high in these types of fibre are wholegrains, legumes, vegetables and fruits.

It is best to get your fibre from eating these wholefoods. Meat, though nutritionally beneficial for other reasons, has no fibre. Fat also has no fibre. Refined foods have had their fibre removed during processing and we know that a diet of refined foods is not only nutrient-depleted but is also devoid of fibre. People who eat a diet mostly consisting of refined foods often experience constipation and are at more risk in developing digestive diseases, heart disease and diabetes. In wholefoods, Nature has given us both kinds of fibre and in the right amounts.

Fibre supplementation

Some people try to compensate for eating a diet of refined foods by adding fibre that has been extracted from its original source. Wheat

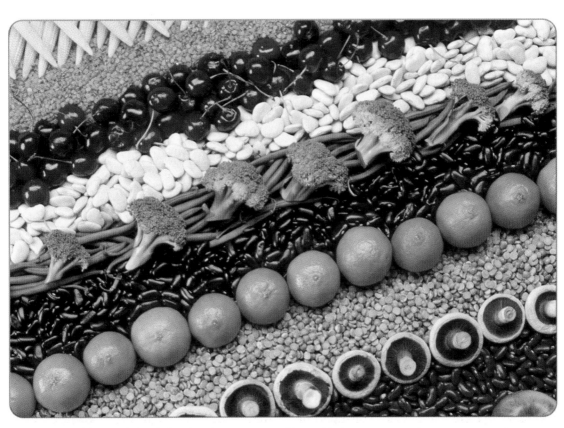

Good sources of fibre include wholegrains, legumes, vegetables and fruits.

bran and oat bran is often sold as fibre supplementation and these are sprinkled on cereals and are added to baked-goods recipes. Since this kind of fibre has been extracted from its original food source, it is not a wholefood. If you use these foods, you might be adding too much of them to your diet and may experience some gas, bloating or digestive distress. Remember that fibre acts like a broom, sweeping the intestine clean of toxins and waste; you want a broom with softer, gentle bristles. Bran by itself can be more like a broom with harsh, scratchy bristles.

There is also some concern that bran alone can deplete the body of minerals. Brans are high in phytic acid, which inhibits the absorption of minerals such as calcium, magnesium and zinc. If you eat a wholegrain, you will be getting its bran along with all its other nutrients.

In a nutshell recipe:

Prune butter; prune and blueberry jam

Nutrition Notes: Prunes are full of fibre and are a good mixture of both insoluble and soluble fibre. The basic prune butter recipe does not have much flavour, but it's a good recipe to add to foods that don't have much fibre. For example, since meat has no fibre, try adding a few tablespoons into a minced meat recipe for making meat loaf.

The prune and blueberry jam variation is delicious. The spices add good flavour to a mixture of fruits that are loaded with antioxidants and are also a good source of fibre.

Basic prune butter

24 organic, unsulphured pitted prunes
175 ml filtered water
Pinch of sea salt

1 In a pan, bring the water to a boil and add the prunes and the sea salt.
2 Simmer, covered, for 3–5 minutes to soften the prunes.
3 Remove from heat and put this mixture in a food processor.
4 Blend well until the mixture has a smooth consistency. (This will take a good 4 minutes or so in the food processor).

Store in an airtight container in the refrigerator. This mixture will keep well for a week in the refrigerator and it also freezes well.

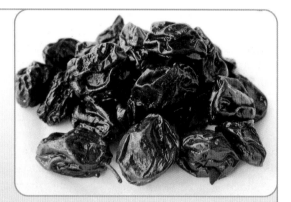

Variation: Prune and blueberry jam

24 organic, unsulphured pitted prunes
65g blueberries
Powdered spices: ⅛ tsp cardamom, ⅛ tsp cinnamon, ¼ tsp ginger, ⅛ tsp allspice
¼ tsp of lemon juice
200 ml of water.

Follow the directions as for basic prune butter, adding the blueberries at Stage 1.

This jam is great with scones. It is delicious on wholemeal toast with almond butter, and with roast pork loin, chicken and turkey, and with roasted sweet potatoes.

Other sources of fibre that you might find in a healthfood store include psyllium seed husks or flaxseeds. I don't recommend the use of psyllium seed husks because many people experience digestive distress with this source of fibre. Flax seeds are a better choice because in addition to providing fibre, these tiny seeds are a source of Omega-3 fatty acids (see Chapter 2) and they have a soothing effect in the intestines.

If you suffer from constipation or any of the other conditions mentioned in this chapter, look at your daily food intake. Do you regularly eat the wholefoods that contain fibre? If not, you may want to consider increasing your consumption of these foods.

The energetic life force in foods

This is a subject you will not see in any traditional book on nutrition. I am presenting it here in an attempt to convince you that a diet of wholefoods is better for your health than a diet of processed refined foods or a diet of fortified foods.

At home I have a vegetable basket into which I put organic vegetables that I have bought at the market. I admit that sometimes there are one or two vegetables that have been in the basket for too long. Typically, these vegetables are carrots, sweet potatoes and onions. What is amazing is that even though these vegetables have been picked out of the earth, transported to market and then taken home to my vegetable basket, they still have the ability to grow. If I keep them in the basket for too long, the carrots grow green tops and white roots, the sweet potatoes grow stems and green leaves and the onions grow green shoots. All of this occurs even though they are no longer planted in the earth and they are not receiving any water! When I see these vegetables, I am reminded of the energy they have within them to continue to grow even though they have been picked from their own source of nourishment.

When we eat a diet of these kinds of foods, we can feel the energy and vibrancy that they have within them. Some food companies are adding vitamins and minerals to their processed foods, such as flaked cereals. These foods are then advertised as being 'fortified' with nutrients. If you count the amounts of specific nutrients of a fortified food, it is even possible to find foods that have higher amounts of these nutrients than do their wholefood equivalents. But in many cases, the nutrients added to the fortified foods are synthetic and are not in the form of vitamins or minerals that our bodies can absorb and use easily.

Try this:

Food experiment

If you are intrigued by the idea of the energetic life force in wholefoods, you could try eating nothing but processed foods for several days, followed by a period of eating nothing but wholefoods for a few days to see if you notice a difference in how you feel on each diet.

Water experiment

Consider the factors mentioned earlier concerning your lifestyle, activity level and the climate you are living in. If you feel you are not drinking enough water, try the following experiment. Increase your daily water intake for a couple of weeks and see if this affects your overall health. Aim to increase your daily water intake to a level where your urine is consistently clear or very light in colour. Record the amount of water it takes per day for you to achieve this quality and make this your water intake for the next few weeks. It should not take you a great amount of water to do this. If you like, try using the idea of the sport bottle with the rubber bands, as Joan did. Keep a record of what you notice about your overall health: Do you feel less tired? Do you feel thirsty at all? Is your skin quality improving? Do you have fewer aches and pains? As time goes on, see if your perception of your water needs increases or decreases and adjust your total amount accordingly.

FAQs

I have heard that I should not drink with meals because it dilutes stomach acid. Is this true?

This is a debatable point. Some nutritionists believe that fluids drunk during meals dilute stomach acid. Some people with digestive problems do find that they digest their food better if they do not drink with meals. But for most people this is not a problem. If you have problems with your digestion, you could try avoiding drinking during meals, and within an hour before and after eating.

What do you think about carbonated or 'fizzy' water?

It is OK to drink carbonated water but you should not have it with meals. Carbonated beverages can neutralize the acid of stomach acid, which you need to help you digest your food, especially the protein portion of your meal.

Might it be dangerous to drink too much water?

People have died from drinking massive amounts of water, but it is rare.

I buy organic wholefood dinners, but they are boxed, frozen and already prepared. What about the nutritional quality of these dinners?

Remember that part of our definition of 'wholefoods' includes foods that are 'prepared in a way that still retains enough nutritional value to be supportive of health'. The fact that your ready-meals are organic is good, but you may want to read the labels to check for added ingredients, such as sugar and salt. As the ready-meals are frozen they will have lost much of their original energetic life force. Therefore, though you can eat them occasionally, it is healthier to plan the majority of your diet to include more fresh wholefoods.

how the body processes food

part three

In this part of *Nutrition In Essence*, you will learn about digestion and detoxification. The ability to digest food well, to assimilate the nutrients from food and then to detoxify any waste products is essential for virtually any health issue. Enhancing digestion and detoxification are two strategies that can have a tremendous positive benefit on overall health.

digestion and detoxification

Impaired digestion is at the heart of most health issues. The process of digestion enables us to absorb the nutrients from our food that we need for all our body functions. You may find that much of the information in this chapter rings bells for you. Hopefully, by the end of the chapter, you will be eager to try some of the strategies to enhance your digestion. Detoxification is another process that enables the body to operate more efficiently. It is all about 'taking out the rubbish'.

Together, digestion and detoxification allow your body to keep the good bits and discard the bad bits. Now let's investigate how your body does this.

Digestion

Some books about nutrition tell you that digestion begins in the mouth. Actually, it begins in your brain. When you see or smell a food that entices you, you may find that you start to salivate. This happens automatically. When you salivate because you have smelled or seen food, your body is preparing to receive food. (In Chapter 7, you will learn that a stressful state shuts down the digestive process.)

The word 'digestion' comes from the Latin *digestio*. It literally means 'to take apart'. If you eat a cucumber sandwich, your body does not need cucumber or bread, it needs the nutrients that the cucumber and bread break down into after you have digested and metabolised them. Your body then uses the nutrients for growth, energy and repair, and eliminates the waste products. The nutrients you get from your food are critical for your survival. They need to be in a form that your body will recognise before it will allow them to be absorbed and used. So, effective digestion is also critical for your survival.

The digestive process

Once you have taken a bite of your cucumber sandwich, the first opportunity you have to turn it into nutrients is by chewing. It may sound simple, but chewing your food well is very important. Digestion is both a mechanical and chemical process. When you chew your food, it mixes with your saliva, which has some digestive enzymes in it. These enzymes and the action of your teeth will start to break down the sandwich before it gets to your stomach. Your grandma was right when she told you not to rush your food.

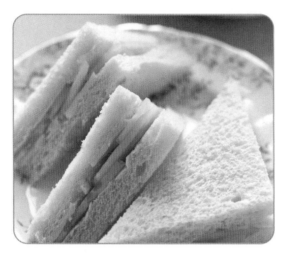

The traditional British cucumber sandwich

After you have chewed well and swallowed a bite of your sandwich, it travels through your oesophagus and reaches your stomach. Your oesophagus is the long tube that connects your mouth to your stomach, and food moves through it in wave-like movements. When your bite of sandwich reaches your stomach it will be further transformed so that it will be in the proper form for your small intestine to receive it. Your small intestine is the place where nutrients from your sandwich are absorbed, so your stomach and the very first part of your small intestine have a lot of work to do.

The stomach

Your stomach has a number of different jobs to do in digesting your sandwich. One of its most important jobs is to sterilise your food. Food comes into your body from the outside world. Stomach acid is so acidic that almost nothing can survive in it. As stomach acid

mixes with your food it kills off any possible pathogen that might have hitched a ride on your sandwich. The digestive enzyme pepsin, which is used in protein digestion, is also produced in the stomach. A very small amount of the digestion of fats occurs in the stomach, but primarily this is where protein digestion really begins. Alcohol is absorbed directly from the stomach into the bloodstream. A substance called intrinsic factor is also produced in the stomach and this substance is necessary for vitamin B12 absorption. Your stomach is also a holding tank: once your food has been sterilised and partly digested, there is a valve at the bottom of your stomach which allows your food to enter the small intestine a little at a time.

The small intestine

When food reaches the point of entry into your small intestine, it is called chyme. As the chyme enters the first part of your small intestine, digestive enzymes from your pancreas and bile from your liver enter via different pathways to join up with the chyme. The digestive enzymes work on all the protein, fats and carbohydrates to digest them even further, and the bile emulsifies the fats so that the digestive enzymes can digest the fats more easily. Emulsifying is what washing-up liquid does to fat and grease on dishes: it breaks up the fat droplets into even smaller droplets. Bile is like washing-up liquid for the fats in your food; it breaks them down into smaller droplets so that the digestive enzyme lipase is able to digest the droplets. Your pancreas also releases sodium bicarbonate, which is highly alkaline. This is necessary to prevent the rest of your digestive tract being burned by the stomach acid in the chyme. Your stomach is not burned because it creates a special substance called mucin that protects the stomach lining from the acid. When the chyme enters the

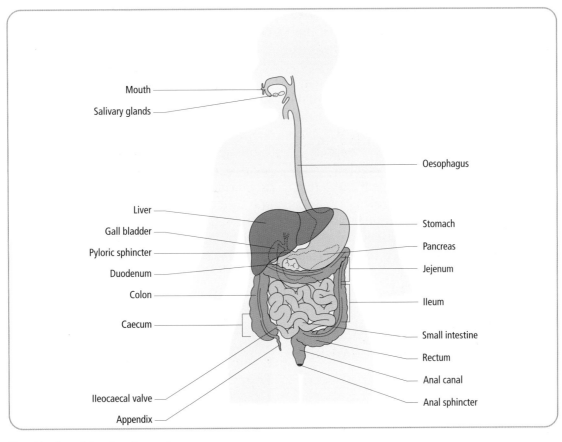

Mouth
Salivary glands
Oesophagus
Liver
Gall bladder
Pyloric sphincter
Duodenum
Colon
Caecum
Stomach
Pancreas
Jejenum
Ileum
Small intestine
Rectum
Anal canal
Anal sphincter
Ileocaecal valve
Appendix

The side view of the digestive system

small intestine, the sodium bicarbonate immediately mixes with it and neutralises the acid. By now, the chyme is in the state it should be in for the nutrients from your original cucumber sandwich to be in particles small enough to pass through the walls of the small intestine into the deeper parts of your body, where they can be used. Anything left over is waste. This passes on through the large intestine and then out through the rectum and anus as faeces. The lining of your small intestine is covered with very small finger-like projections called villi, which cover it like a velvety forest. As the nutrients pass through the villi forest, the villi usher them in and they are absorbed through the wall of the intestine. The tips of the villi also contain the enzyme lactase, which helps you to digest lactose, the sugar that is found in milk. Good villi health is extremely important for digestion. (In Chapter 11 you will learn about a specific food sensitivity that destroys villi.) Once the remains of the chyme are through your small intestine, they move into your large intestine – the colon.

The colon

Your colon has a set of functions. Here, fluid left in the remaining chyme is absorbed through the colon walls as water for your body to use. Your colon is also home to a variety of different species of flora: mostly bacteria. Roughly two kilos of your body weight are the flora that lives in your colon. Considering that bacteria are tiny creatures, you can imagine how many of them are living inside you. If this idea makes you squeamish, it is important to remember that good bacteria are your friends because they work hard to keep you healthy. Good bacteria help you to fight infection, produce some B-vitamins and keep away the bad bacteria. These friendly bacteria also help increase your resistance to food poisoning, recycle bile salts, help to regulate your immune system, provide nutrition that nourishes the lining of your intestinal walls (a fatty acid that is also found in butter) and may even suppress tumors. That is a lot of work for these tiny creatures to do. Bad bacteria create toxins that your hard-working liver must then detoxify.

When a baby is born, its intestines are sterile and ready to be populated with flora. Breast milk is the best choice for baby's nourishment in this case because mother's milk introduces good healthy flora into the baby's system. For women who cannot breastfeed, Sally Fallon has some wonderful recipes for baby formula in her book *Nourishing Traditions*.

It is best to avoid soya-based formulas because the isoflavones in soy have too strong an oestrogenic effect on an infant's developing endocrine system.

In a nutshell recipe:

Cooking perfect grains

Chapter 1 explains how soaking grains, beans and legumes with the juice of half a lemon overnight or for eight hours can make them more digestible. Here is another tip to help you cook perfect grains. This example shows how to prevent brown rice becoming stodgy and lumpy. After washing and soaking the rice, drain the soaking water and add filtered water for cooking. Japanese people eat a lot of rice and this is how they prepare it. Many Japanese cooks don't measure the amount of water, they just add water up to the level of the first crease in the second finger, when the finger is placed on top of the rice. Add a pinch of sea salt. Cover the pan and bring it to a boil on high heat. As soon as it boils, lower the heat and simmer the rice until the water seems to have almost disappeared. Do not stir the rice while it is cooking. Remove the pan from the heat and place a tea towel under the lid of the pan. Let the rice steam itself until cooked. When you are ready to serve it, fluff the rice gently with a wooden spoon. Do not stir.

The tea towel under the pot lid is a Japanese cooking technique. If you don't use a tea towel at this point, the water condenses on the lid of

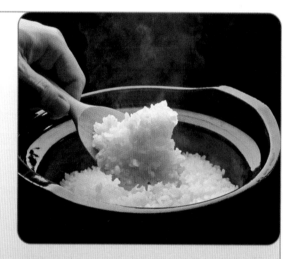

the pan and falls back onto the rice. This makes the rice stodgy. The tea towel absorbs the steam.

Additional tip: If you are not cooking on a gas flame, use two burners and start with one on high heat and then move the pan quickly to the other which is on low heat. This will simulate cooking on gas. Always use a good-quality heavy pan when cooking grains so that the grains won't burn on the bottom of the pan.

Taking steps to enhance your digestion is the most important nutritional strategy you can employ to achieve better health. There are recommendations on how to enhance your digestion at the end of this chapter.

Detoxification

Every day we face toxicity: it comes from the environment, from pathogens, from chemicals we breathe in or eat, drugs, and even from the by-products of our own metabolic processes. No matter how careful we are, we can't avoid all toxins.

In America, in 2003, the Environmental Working Group (EWG) tested the blood and urine of nine volunteers and discovered 167 industrial and chemical pollutants in their blood, some of which were carcinogenic. None of the people tested worked in industrial or chemical industries. The EWG calls the cocktail of toxins that we are exposed to as our 'body burden'.

We have little control over our exposure to these chemicals. If we add to this burden the toxicity from lifestyle factors over which we do have some control, such as drug use; the consumption of foods with pesticides, food additives and colourings; smoking, sugar, alcohol and artificial sweeteners, we can begin to imagine the burden we are putting on our bodies' detoxification systems.

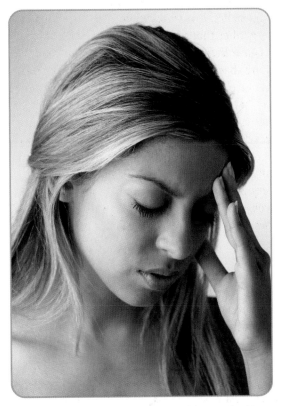

A high body burden of toxins can result in poor health

The liver

The liver is the major detoxification organ in the body and has a tremendous job to do.

You've got to love your liver. It performs many functions for you, including filtering and cleaning your blood, converting thyroid hormones, breaking down old hormones and creating new ones, making proteins, making bile, storing some nutrients and detoxifying toxins. (Symptoms of a toxic, overworked liver include migraines, eczema, skin rashes, fatigue and allergies.)

The two phases of detoxification

When your liver detoxifies a substance, it does so in two phases, appropriately named Phase I and Phase II. Phase I involves a lot of enzymes, which turn a toxin into a water-soluble form or into a more chemically active form. Phase 1 occurs in the liver but also elsewhere in the body; especially places where toxins may enter. If the toxin becomes water-soluble, then it can be eliminated through your kidneys in your urine. If the toxin becomes more metabolically active, then it becomes more poisonous. It seems odd that the liver should turn a toxin into something even more poisonous than the original one, but it does this because that is the form the toxin must be in to go through Phase II. However, in this intermediate stage, the converted toxin has time to do some damage. Therefore it is important to have good liver health so that both phases are working well.

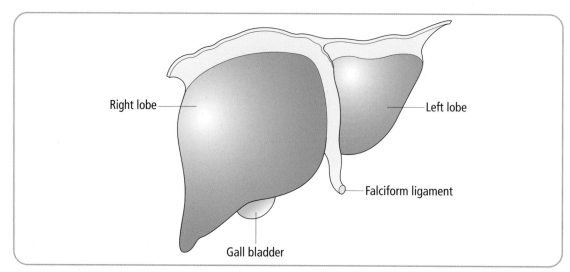

Right lobe

Left lobe

Falciform ligament

Gall bladder

The liver

The intermediate stage is the reason why poisonous mushrooms can kill you. If you eat one, your liver will attempt to detoxify the toxin from the mushroom by first undergoing Phase I. In doing so, the liver makes an intermediate substance that is very damaging to its own cells. In this case, cell death can be so extensive that it kills you.

After the intermediate stage, the converted toxin is sent to Phase II. In Phase II, your liver conjugates, or joins chemicals to the toxin. This either renders the toxin totally harmless or converts it into a form that can be excreted through the urine or through the bile that the liver also creates.

Sources of toxicity

Though the idea of 'body burden' may seem bleak, there are some sources of toxicity that you can try to avoid. Cigarette smoke, excess alcohol, sugar, drugs, excess caffeine, artificial sweeteners, food additives and pesticides found on processed and non-organic foods all create toxicity – some more than others. Often, we can choose to avoid many of these substances. Heavy metal exposure is another source of toxicity. Heavy metals include mercury, lead and cadmium. You can be exposed to these through the environment, the 'silver' fillings in your teeth, cigarette smoking, old building paint (which may contain lead) and other sources. There is some concern that

fatty fish, though good for you in terms of their fat content, may be contaminated with mercury, especially the larger fish.

Heavy metals can affect your health negatively. They can displace other beneficial minerals from your body. The best way to rid them from your body is to reduce exposure if you can and then to eat foods that chelate them. Chelation means that substances in these foods will bind to the heavy metals and take them out of your body. Eating an organic wholefood diet that includes leafy greens and some raw nuts and seeds can help provide your body with the nutrients it needs to help rid it of toxicity.

In a nutshell recipe:

Powerful pesto

This pesto is delicious and contains liver-enhancing foods. Parsley is a leafy green full of good antioxidants. The nuts and seeds contain even more antioxidants such as selenium, and vitamin E and beneficial minerals such as magnesium and zinc. Raw garlic is well known for its antifungal and antibiotic qualities, and sea salt provides more trace minerals. Though the taste of this pesto will entice you, eat this as a 'wholefood helper' – so not too much at a time! Use organic ingredients.

16 shelled raw Brazil nuts
30g shelled raw sunflower seeds
35g raw pumpkin seeds
1 medium clove garlic, chopped

1 medium bunch of fresh Italian flat-leaf parsley, leaves only
1 medium bunch of fresh basil leaves
75 ml extra virgin olive oil
1 tbsp lemon juice
¼ tsp sea salt

1 Process the nuts, seeds and garlic in a food processor until well ground.
2 Add parsley, basil, lemon juice, salt and olive oil. Process until the mixture is well blended and starts to form a ball in the food processor.
3 To thin out, add 2 tbsns water.

Keep in an airtight container in the fridge. It also freezes well. Use as a condiment for fish, meat or chicken. You can also add it to grain salads or put it on jacket potatoes. For a snack, stuff into a few celery sticks.

How toxins affect hormones

There are toxins in the environment that have a direct impact on our hormones. They are hormone-like substances that act in a similar way to human hormones when they enter the body. Though modern life has given us many conveniences, it has also given us substances that never existed in nature but that we are exposed to. Xeno-oestrogens are foreign substances that are not real oestrogen but act like it. These are chemicals found in substances like plastics and pesticides. If you microwave food that has clingfilm wrap over it and the food is touching the clingfilm, or if you eat food that has been sprayed with pesticides, you may be taking in xeno-oestrogens. Researchers believe that even though they are not real oestrogen, their effect in the body is to add to your total oestrogen level. This is a problem because oestrogen should be in balance with progesterone. The balance exists in the ratio between the two hormones, not their levels. If you have a higher amount of oestrogen compared to your progesterone you are in oestrogen dominance. Even if you are a woman in menopause and you have low oestrogen levels, you can still have oestrogen dominance because your progesterone levels are also low so the ratio of oestrogen to progesterone is still higher. Oestrogen dominance can put a woman at risk of developing oestrogen-dependent cancers such as breast cancer. (Read more about this topic in Chapter 9.) It is your liver's task to take apart and detoxify xeno-oestrogens. Supporting the health of your liver is critical for your overall good health.

Digestive conditions

Some of the conditions associated with the digestive and detoxification system include:

- heartburn
- constipation
- irritable bowel syndrome (IBS)
- gallstones.

61

Heartburn

Heartburn occurs when stomach acid backs up into the oesophagus, causing a burning sensation. Smoking, alcohol consumption, food sensitivities, overeating, fried foods, dehydration and inadequate chewing can contribute to heartburn problems. Mostly, if you consume a plant-based diet of whole foods, you can avoid heartburn because these foods tend to be alkalising, rather than acidic.

Constipation

Constipation happens when faecal matter remains in the colon for too long a period of time. Though it can be caused by a medical problem such as colon obstruction or as a side effect of some drugs, it is far more commonly a problem of poor food choices. It is very important to have fibre in your diet. You will naturally have more fibre in your diet if you eat more wholefoods. Refined foods have been stripped of their fibre. Dehydration can also be a factor in constipation. Regular exercise is also helpful.

Irritable bowel syndrome (IBS)

IBS occurs when the colon is not working properly and it becomes inflamed. There can be abdominal pain, nausea, loss of appetite and either constipation or diarrhoea. IBS is often linked to stress. The state of your nervous system affects your digestion profoundly and this has a significant impact on its functioning: You may have heard the expressions 'butterflies in the stomach' or 'gut feelings'. In Chapter 7 and Chapter 11 you can read more about the impact that stress and food intolerances have on your digestive system. Employing stress-management techniques and following the guidelines below for enhancing your digestion can help alleviate IBS.

Gallstones

The bile that your liver makes carries fat-soluble toxins into your lower digestive tract for elimination. Your gall bladder stores bile for when it is needed. Gallstones can block the flow of this bile. A diet of bad fats, low fibre and a lack of alkalising foods such as fruits and vegetables can contribute to the formation of gallstones.

Enhancing your digestion

Taking steps to improve your digestion and to have a healthy liver are the most important positive nutritional activities you can undertake towards better health. Here are some dietary and lifestyle suggestions for enhancing your digestion and supporting your liver:

- Follow the general guidelines for a healthier diet as outlined in Chapter 1.

- Eat organic food as much as possible. The residue of pesticides on non-organic produce is toxins. It can't always be removed by washing. Organic food is Genetically Modified (GM) free. Emphasise sulphur-rich foods, which include garlic, onions, and eggs. These assist the liver's detoxification pathways. Other foods that assist the liver include leafy greens and other vegetables: broccoli, cauliflower, Brussels sprouts, cabbage, artichoke, asparagus and avocado.

- Remember to chew your food well and take time to eat. Try to calm yourself before you eat a meal.

- If you are unused to chewing or if you have difficulty in digesting your food, cut your food into very small bites or include more soups and puréed food in your diet. This might be especially beneficial for elderly people or people who have been ill.

- If you are going to use fats in cooking, choose butter, ghee, coconut oil or olive oil. Heat the pan before adding the fat or oil and have everything ready to add to the pan. This minimises the amount of time the food stays in the heated pan. Stir-frying, boiling, steaming and baking are good methods of cooking. Frying results in foods that are tougher on the digestion. See Chapter 2 for a discussion on good fats and bad fats.

- Try to get sugar out of your diet. It upsets the balance of healthy intestinal flora. It also feeds pathogenic bacteria. Also avoid refined foods, as they have little nutritional value.

- Enhance protein digestion by introducing 'bitters' or a 'digestive' before a meal. Many cultures of the world do this as a matter of course.

- Soak all grains and beans and legumes overnight or for at least eight hours before cooking. Refer to the guidelines in Chapters 1 and 5 for preparing and cooking beans, legumes and grains.

- Add fermented foods such as live yogurt, kefir, natural miso or natural sauerkraut to your diet. This will encourage the growth of the good bacteria in your intestines.

- Try not to overuse over-the-counter antacids. They counteract your stomach acid which you need to sterilise your food, to help with protein digestion and to allow absorption of vitamin B12. Most people will find that if they enhance their digestion, they won't need antacids.

- Identify any food intolerances you have and avoid these foods. (See Chapter 11).

- There are many herbs that can be extremely useful in digestion and detoxification. Silymarin, or milk thistle, is very protective for your liver. In animal studies, it has even been protective against the destruction caused by ingestion of poisonous mushrooms. Consult with a herbalist for a recommendation of which herbs to include in your diet and how to use milk thistle.

FAQs

I have been told that we must practice food combining to have the best digestion. Is this a good idea?

There are some people who benefit from food combining, but mostly I believe they are benefiting from shifting their diet from one of refined processed foods to a more wholefood diet, which food combining also indirectly encourages. Food combining principles ask you to eat fast-fermenting fruits like berries and melons alone, not to mix animal proteins with starches and to eat only carbohydrate foods at breakfast. Other advice includes avoiding refined carbohydrates and basically to eat a diet based largely on plants. I have found that if most people follow a wholefood diet, identify any food intolerances they have and follow steps to enhance their digestion, they don't need food combining. Dietary practices that make you have to think too much about food preparation are not practical. Most cultures across the world have a traditional chicken and rice dish, which as it mixes animal protein with a starch is contrary to food combining principles. Business travellers who cross time zones will often find it difficult to determine when 'morning' is in order to eat only carbohydrates then. Most indigenous healthy cultures around the world don't practise limiting or specific diets; they eat the foods that are available to them.

What do you think about fasting as a plan for detoxification?

The practice of fasting, or avoiding food for a period of time, is an ancient one. Fasting gives the digestive system a rest and allows your body to cleanse itself. However, this is really only appropriate for someone who is in a good enough state of health to handle it. I don't advocate fasting for anyone who has very low energy, is depleted or needs to rebuild their body. I have seen very toxic-laden people go on fasts and start to feel miserable within 24 hours. They may be told that feeling bad is a good thing, because they are experiencing a 'healing crisis', but what is really happening is that the toxicity that has been liberated from their cells is still travelling around in their bloodstream. Also, the body burden that we are all exposed to today makes fasting more of a problem unless we have already maximized our digestion and worked on making our livers healthier. I feel it is best to get on a healthy diet first and to achieve a level of health and vibrancy before you consider any kind of a fast. If you do decide to fast and you have not done so before, it is best to do it with the help of a practitioner who is experienced in working with people who are fasting.

I have heard that raw foods are best to eat because they retain all their nutrients and enzymes and that cooking destroys nutrients. Is this true?

Yes and No. Heat destroys some vitamins and phytonutrients. The amount of nutrients that are destroyed through cooking depends on the method of cooking and for how long the foods are cooked. Stir-frying, steaming, poaching, baking and boiling for a short period of time are the best methods of cooking. For vegetables, the best approach is to cook them just until their colour is more vibrant, and no longer. Raw foods do retain their nutrients. However, some people have a difficult time digesting raw foods. For these people, light cooking is better because the cooking 'predigests' the food. Also, the enzymes that are present in raw foods are not the same as our own digestive enzymes. Some nutrients are actually enhanced through cooking. For example, the amounts of the phytonutrient lycopene is increased in tomatoes when they are cooked. The best overall strategy is to eat a variety of foods that have been prepared in a variety of ways.

nutritional issues

part four

This section of *Nutrition in Essence* introduces you to wholefood nutrition and a range of health conditions. Here you will learn how wholefood nutrition principles can be applied to specific health conditions. You will also learn how to incorporate more specific nutrition suggestions into your overall healthier diet.

blood sugar

'Why am I so tired?' This is a question I hear a lot from my clients. Many doctors say that fatigue is the reason why most of their patients consult them. Once medical reasons for fatigue (such as anaemia or hypothyroid) have been ruled out by your doctor, the commonest reason for fatigue is blood-sugar dysregulation. This chapter looks at blood sugar and how it relates to fatigue, and at one of the major health issues facing society today: diabetes.

How insulin works

In Chapter 2 you learned about carbohydrates. When you eat foods that are primarily carbohydrate, they metabolise to a sugar called glucose. When we think of carbohydrates as our major source of energy, the energy source is really glucose. This is the only form of sugar that your body can utilise. After the carbohydrates you have eaten have been metabolised into glucose, this sugar enters your bloodstream. But glucose cannot be used for energy while it is in your blood. It is only on a journey and needs to reach its intended destination. It must be taken out of the bloodstream and put into your cells where it can be burned as energy. The only way it can do this is to have the hormone insulin present. Insulin acts as a carrier and escorts glucose into your cells. Without insulin, glucose cannot get into your cells. It is almost as if the inside of the cells is an exclusive club and the

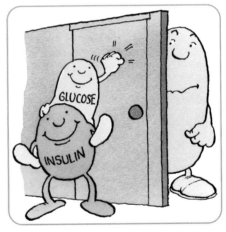

Glucose must be with insulin to get through the cell "door"

club will only allow glucose to enter if insulin escorts it in. Without insulin, the receptor site acts like a 'bouncer' at the cell membrane entrance and tells glucose: 'No, you can't come in. You must have insulin with you!' This is the problem that diabetics have.

'Type 1' diabetes

People with Type 1 Diabetes either cannot make insulin or they cannot make enough of it. Type 1 diabetics are insulin-dependent and must get it from an outside source, usually in the form of insulin injections. Type 1 Diabetes is usually diagnosed early in childhood or by young adulthood and because of this it is referred to as 'juvenile-onset diabetes'. We don't really know the reason why people have this disease, but it is thought to be due to an autoimmune condition where the person's own immune system attacks and destroys the cells of the pancreas that produce insulin. In such a case, the immune system believes that these cells are harmful pathogens and does not recognise them as part of the body.

'Type 2' diabetes

Type 1 Diabetes is not the most common form of diabetes. In recent years our society has seen the rise of Type 2 Diabetes and this form is currently almost at epidemic levels. With Type 2 Diabetes, the cells of the pancreas are able to make insulin, but the entrance of glucose plus insulin into the cells that need the glucose for energy is blocked. In this case, it is as if glucose and insulin are knocking on the entrance door of the cell but the 'bouncer' has earphones on and cannot hear them, so the door to the cell remains closed. Type 2 Diabetes usually occurs after years of poor dietary habits and can therefore be prevented through diet. This is the good news. The bad news is that it used to be called 'adult-onset diabetes' because it did not occur in people until their adult years, but it is no longer called this because cases of Type 2 Diabetes are developing in children as young as ten years of age. Why is this happening?

Diet and diabetes

As a society we are now consuming greater amounts of sugar and refined carbohydrates than ever before. Sugar and refined-carbohydrate foods are fast-releasing glucose foods and so they are metabolised very quickly by the body. With these kinds of foods in your diet, you are dumping large amounts of glucose into your bloodstream at once.

Your body is designed to eat a wholefood diet, as our ancestors did when they were foraging for food and eating wholefoods such as leafy greens, nuts, seeds, berries and, occasionally, wild game and fish. These kinds of foods are slow-releasing glucose foods because they are metabolised slowly. With these kinds of foods in your diet you are slowly feeding glucose into your bloodstream.

Diet and blood sugar

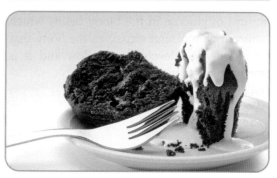
Refined carbohydrates

Today's food choices offer many varieties of packaged and processed foods and most of these are refined foods. Whereas we used to drink water, we now drink fizzy drinks, fruit juices and drinks that contain large amounts of sugar. Whether you consume a wholefood diet or you consume a diet full of sugar and refined carbohydrates, your body will respond to your dietary choices by producing the hormones and enzymes necessary to metabolise your food and drink choices for as long as it can. Your dietary choices will determine whether you are nourishing your body or putting a stress on it to metabolise foods and drinks that call for large amounts of hormones and enzymes.

Fluctuation of blood sugar levels

In the Blood Sugar Diagrams depicted overleaf, you will see examples of a person's blood-sugar levels throughout a one-day timeline. Diagram 1 shows two lines: a hypothetical upper limit for blood-sugar levels and a hypothetical lower limit for blood-sugar levels. The upper limit is the amount of glucose in the blood beyond which the brain would send signals to the pancreas to make insulin because it senses the rise in glucose after the person has eaten some food with carbohydrate. The lower limit represents the amount of glucose in the blood below which the brain would send signals to the body that the blood-sugar levels are too low and it is time to make them rise again. In this case, the signals would be hunger, or cravings to eat more carbohydrates.

Food choices and blood sugar

Diagrams 2 and 3 in Figure 6.3 show the impact that food choice has on blood-sugar levels as the body is called upon to produce the hormone insulin.

Good food choices

Diagram 2 shows a day of eating wholefoods, where there is a gradual rise in blood sugar and insulin is produced accordingly. The insulin escorts the glucose into the cells for energy. The blood-sugar level falls and does not rise until the person eats a wholefood carbohydrate again. When they do, the same pattern occurs. This picture is a healthy one, showing a situation where the person is not skipping meals, is eating healthy foods and the body is managing the slow metabolism of carbohydrates well. On the left side of the timeline, which represents morning, you will notice that the person's blood-sugar levels are somewhat low because the person did not eat at night. Breakfast is the first meal of the day and the word breakfast means just that: it is breaking the fast of the previous night. Breakfast is the most important meal of the day. It sets up your blood-sugar picture for the rest of the day by helping you to stay out of a low blood-sugar trough. Choosing wholefoods for breakfast as this person did allows your body to metabolise the carbohydrate part of the meal more slowly and release glucose into the bloodstream in a slow but steady pattern.

Poor food choices

Diagram 3 does not show a healthy picture. Here, the person is probably eating refined carbohydrates and sugar, which are being metabolised very quickly. This makes blood-sugar levels also rise quickly, as the glucose is released into the blood in large amounts at once. Here, you see a roller-coaster effect: after the initial huge rise in blood sugar, the pancreas is called upon to make the amount of insulin that can move the large amount of glucose out of the blood and into the cells. But the time-lag involved makes for a corresponding huge drop in blood-sugar levels as all the glucose is moved out.

Blood Sugar Diagrams

Diagram 1: A picture of the upper and lower acceptable limits of blood-sugar levels on a one-day timeline.

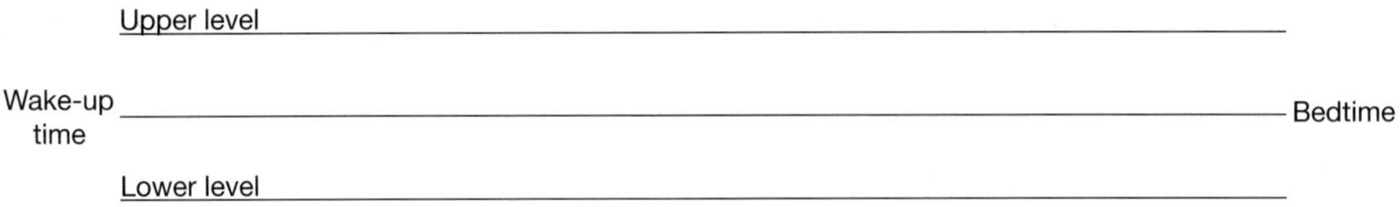

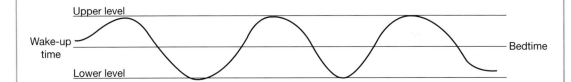

Diagram 2: A picture of diagram 1 above, with a wavy line showing how the body would like its blood-sugar levels to be. (Maybe more like what our caveperson ancestors' blood-sugar picture would have been).

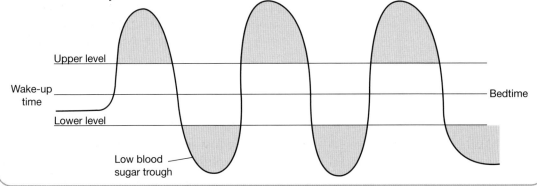

Diagram 3: A picture of diagram 1, large wavy line showing how many of today's populations' blood-sugar picture most likely looks. This is a strain on the body's function and takes its toll over time.

The trough that you see below the 'acceptable' line is a situation called hypoglycaemia, or low blood sugar. If you have ever been in a low blood-sugar trough, you do not feel well. You might feel exhausted, shaky, irritable, depressed, anxious, teary or extremely hungry and you might also crave sugar or other carbohydrates. Your body is not designed to handle large amounts of glucose but it will when called upon to do so. On the left side of this timeline, you will notice that the person's blood-sugar level is very low when they wake up. This is because they did not eat at night, but with poor food choices the day before, they have more of a tendency to be in a low blood-sugar trough when they wake. If this is your typical picture, you may also be one of those people who crave sugary or refined food first thing in the morning. Your body is responding to its very low blood sugar. This is the main reason that some people crave sugar, while others do not.

If you consistently choose foods and drinks that are high in sugar or refined carbohydrates, your pancreas will become tired of having to make such large amounts of insulin and it will become less able to do so as time goes on, unless you change your diet. Over time, you will also feel an overall level of fatigue. This establishment of habitual poor blood-sugar control is the most common reason for fatigue that I see in my clients. Once they switch from eating sugar and refined foods to a wholefood diet they find that their energy levels rise, they become less moody or irritable and they lose cravings for sugar.

Eating regularly

Timing of eating is also an important consideration in managing blood-sugar levels. Another typical pattern I see in my clients is one of skipping breakfast, sometimes skipping lunch and then eating a huge dinner followed by a very sugary dessert. With this pattern there is also a tendency to crave sugar, especially in the late afternoon. The blood sugar diagram illustrates the effects this eating pattern has on blood-sugar levels. If you eat this way, it is stressful for your body because you will be in a low blood-sugar trough for most of the day and then when you eat foods that are high in sugar, you will again get the high blood-sugar 'spike' followed by the low blood-sugar 'crash'. With this pattern, you are depriving your body of the good nutrition it needs throughout the day to fuel your body and stressing your pancreas by forcing it to produce large amounts of insulin in short periods of time. If this is your blood-sugar picture, you will probably feel fatigued for most of the day and ravenous in the evening. You may also crave sugar and/or caffeine because of your low energy levels.

Taking control of your blood sugar

Type 2 Diabetes is really the end of a continuum of blood-sugar dysregulation. Though it may seem so to people who have been diagnosed as diabetics, they do not wake up one morning as a diabetic having not been one the day before. The diagnosis may seem sudden, but really it is the result of years of blood-sugar dysregulation. Many of us have just got used to feeling tired and having low levels of energy, believing that it is just a normal part of life. Taking steps to control your blood-sugar levels can have a profound effect on your overall sense of wellbeing.

The first step is to ensure that we are trying to establish a picture of healthy blood-sugar levels throughout each day. Although Type 2 Diabetes is a disease that is predominantly caused by a long period of poor eating habits and reversing these habits can, in some cases, reverse diabetes, there is a point of no return. When the disease has progressed to a point where there is death of the cells in the pancreas that produce insulin, Type 2 Diabetes can become insulin-dependent Type 1 Diabetes. This is a new health phenomenon. Given the fact that we are also seeing Type 2 Diabetes develop in children, this does not bode well for the future of our children unless we intervene and change their diets. If we do not, as grim as this sounds, we may be the first generation to outlive our children.

The glycaemic index (GI)

To help consumers identify which foods are the healthiest in maintaining stable blood-sugar levels, researchers have created the glycaemic index of foods. This is an index that compares the body's glucose response to the carbohydrates in individual foods against the glucose response to a reference food. There are different glycaemic index (GI) charts: some compare the glucose response of foods against the glucose response of white bread and some compare the glucose response of foods against the glucose response of glucose itself. The higher the GI number a food has, the more rapid a glucose response the body has against that food. It was thought that if people had this list of foods with glycaemic numbers, they could design their diets around foods that had lower GI numbers and therefore be able to balance their blood-sugar levels easily. If a food has been given a number of 70 or above, it is a high-glycaemic-response food.

GI cautions

The glycaemic index is presented here because you will most likely read about it in other books and magazine articles. However, there are some problems with the glycaemic index. Because of the way that foods are compared, it is only the carbohydrate content of the food that is considered. Therefore, if the reference food is glucose at 100 grams and the food being compared to the glucose is 100 grams of carbohydrate of that food, the index can make a healthy food that does not have a lot of carbohydrate in it look 'bad'. You may recall

from Chapter 2 that most foods are not made up of only one nutrient. This can make the glycaemic index skewed against wholefoods because you would need to eat a huge and unrealistic amount of the food to get 100 grams of carbohydrate from it, and yet the number that food is given on the glycaemic index is high. For example, on one glycaemic index list, carrots have a GI number of 92 while Mars Bars have a GI number of 91! Clearly, it is not realistic to compare the health values of carrots with Mars Bars in this way.

Another problem with the glycaemic index is that it traditionally compares foods against glucose. Therefore other sugars may not have an index rating reflective of how they are metabolised in the body. For example, fructose, the sugar found in fruit, has a GI number of 0. This might make you think that fructose is a really healthy sugar to use. If you are eating a piece of fruit, such as an apple, it can be. But you can also get processed fructose as a sugar substitute in many healthfood stores. Fructose may not elevate insulin levels and this control mechanism of blood sugar has been the primary point of discussion here, but fructose has other problems associated with its use. The liver rapidly assimilates fructose. Through its metabolic pathways, fructose can contribute to elevated triglycerides and cholesterol. The natural fructose that is found in whole foods, such that found in an apple, can be healthy because it exists in amounts that are balanced with the other nutrients found in the apple, such as the fibre, which will slow down the metabolism of the fructose. Processed fructose, sold as a diabetic alternative to sugar, is not a healthy option. The absolute worse form of fructose is high fructose corn syrup. This is a highly processed form of fructose that is in fizzy drinks and fruit drinks as well as a sweetener in many processed foods.

Another problem with the glycaemic index is that foods are analysed as if they are eaten alone. In reality, people eat a variety of foods together in a meal and the nutrient content of all foods eaten will have an impact on overall blood-sugar levels. Therefore, if you eat carrots that are in a stew along with meat and other vegetables and some olive oil, the carrot will not affect your overall blood sugar levels adversely.

Glycaemic load

This involves a calculation designed to take into consideration the basic premise of the glycaemic index (how much of an influence the food's carbohydrates have on blood-sugar levels) but it also considers the quality of the food being consumed. Carrots might then stand a better chance at being rated as a healthier option to Mars Bars with the glycaemic load rating! Following a wholefood diet will naturally meet the goals of consuming low-glycaemic-load foods. The important thing to keep in mind is that eating a varied wholefood diet will automatically help to balance your blood-sugar levels.

In a nutshell recipe:

South Indian spiced roasted root vegetables

Nutrition Notes: This recipe calls for vegetables that are higher in carbohydrates, but it can really help someone to transition off refined carbohydrate foods and sugar. When you roast root vegetables, their natural sweetness is enhanced. In addition to their sweetness, vegetables have many nutrients that make them much healthier choices than refined foods. As far as possible, choose organic vegetables for this recipe.

---

1 medium swede
1 medium turnip
2 parsnips
2 carrots
(Peel and chop all the vegetables into 1-inch and half-inch chunks)
¼ tsp sea salt
¼ tsp cumin powder
¼ tsp teaspoon turmeric powder
Pinch of red chilli pepper flakes (optional)
1 tbsp coconut oil, melted

1 Peel and chop the vegetables into 1-inch and half-inch chunks. Make sure all the vegetable pieces are roughly the same size so they will be ready at the same time.

2 If it is hard at room temperature, warm the coconut oil until just melted and remove from heat.
3 Put the dry spices into a plastic bag (a sandwich bag that seals is good for this). Add the melted coconut oil and the vegetables.
4 Seal the bag and shake it well to coat the vegetables with the spices and the coconut oil. Work quickly, because as the coconut oil cools down it will become less liquid.
5 Tip the mixture out onto a baking sheet that has been lined with greaseproof baking paper.
6 Roast in a hot oven (425 degrees Fahrenheit/210 degrees Celsius) for 15 minutes or until just tender when pricked with a fork. Use an oven rack placed in the middle of the oven to prevent the vegetables from burning.

Mediterranean Variation: use the same vegetables and the sea salt, but replace the coconut oil, cumin, turmeric and chilli pepper with:
1 tbsp olive oil
¼ tsp of dried thyme
¼ tsp of dried sage
¼ tspn dried, crushed rosemary
Follow the same cooking directions.

casestudy: Sleepy Sue

Sue was a client aged 62 who had recently been diagnosed with Type 2 Diabetes. She complained of extreme fatigue. In fact, hers was the worst case of fatigue I have ever seen – Sue said she often fell asleep at the wheel while driving! Her Dietary and Lifestyle (DAL) record (see the next page) showed that she ate a lot of gluten, grains and refined carbohydrates, some protein and very little fat. Her doctor had said that she needed to lose weight and told her to avoid fat in her diet. Through testing, we discovered that she was gluten-intolerant and Sue agreed to avoid it. She also agreed to maintain her dietary intake records and to replace all her refined foods with wholefoods. She decided to stay off grains altogether and to use vegetables as her sources of carbohydrates. She ate protein at every meal and included the healthy fats. Sue's was a remarkable success story. Within two weeks her energy levels rose and she no longer felt sleepy while driving. Within a month, her doctor told her she was no longer diabetic.

Keeping blood sugar stable

Here are some dietary and lifestyle suggestions for keeping blood sugar levels stable. You will find a blank copy of a Dietary and Lifestyle (DAL) form on the next page. The DAL is where you can record your intake of food and drink, the time of day you eat, the exercise you get, your lifestyle activities and how you feel throughout the day. If you are diligent about keeping these records, you can learn a lot about how nutrition and lifestyle affect how you feel. You can also look for patterns to see if certain foods affect how you feel.

First, use your DAL record to record several days of your eating and activity habits. Look for answers to the following questions:

- Is there a significant amount of sugar or refined foods in your diet?

- Do you drink fruit juices or drinks?

- Do you skip meals or are there periods of time longer than three or four hours that you go without eating anything?

- Do you notice times of day when you feel fatigued, irritable, sad, shaky or weak and can you look back and associate these times with skipping meals?

If you answered 'Yes' to any of these questions, here are some suggestions for better blood sugar balance:

- Follow the general guidelines for a healthier diet as outlined in Chapter 1.

- Do not skip meals, especially breakfast.

- Eat something every 3–4 hours. Neither your meals nor your snacks need be large.

- Having some protein at every meal will help to balance blood-sugar levels. It does not have to be much: for example, it can be a piece of fish the size of the palm of your hand, two eggs, half a tin of tuna fish, 100 grams of beans or of cottage cheese.

- The mineral chromium is helpful in maintaining blood-sugar levels. Foods higher in chromium include meats, nuts, shellfish and wholegrains.

Dietary and Lifestyle (DAL) Record
(Use one page per day)

Name: _____ Date: _____

Time	Food or drink consumed	Exercise taken	How I felt today (moods, emotions, symptoms, temperature)

- Limit fruits in your diet and avoid dried fruits as these are concentrated in sugar. Have no more than two pieces of fruit per day and eat some protein or healthy fat with them. For example, apple slices with cottage cheese or apple slices with almond butter.

- Include healthy fats in your diet and avoid unhealthy fats. (Refer to Chapter 2 for more information on fats.) If you can find it, coconut oil is very beneficial and can increase metabolism. It is also supportive of thyroid health and therefore can be very energising for those who feel fatigue. Aim for 2–3 tablespoons per day and use it in cooking or drizzle it over steamed vegetables. (Try the recipe in this chapter).

- If you are sedentary, try to bring some form of exercise into your life. The best form of exercise for balancing blood sugar is exercise that builds toned muscles – and no, you need not become a 'bodybuilder'. Toned muscle is more metabolically active and enhances blood-sugar maintenance. If you need to, consult with a fitness expert.

FAQs

My DAL records show that I have a lot of refined carbohydrates in my diet and not much fat or protein. I also use sugar. I have got used to making ready-made meals that are quick and easy to prepare because I am very busy. I want to change my diet but I'm afraid of doing this too suddenly. What should I do?

This is a very good question! To change a diet that is high in refined carbohydrate suddenly can cause even more fatigue while your body adjusts. Keep your intake records every day and make small changes. Start by not skipping meals, especially breakfast, and by making sure you have some protein at every meal.

I drink a lot of soft drinks and fruit juices and I would like to switch to drinking more water, but I'm afraid I'll miss the juice. What should I do?

The same advice for the previous question applies here. Switch gradually. Also, you might try the Vital Vegetable Broth in Chapter 1 to replace some of your drinks. It is naturally sweet because of the root vegetables, but also has the minerals from the vegetables that will help to alkalise your body as it recovers from eating a diet that is acidifying.

I like a glass of wine for dinner every night. Do I have to give that up?

Alcohol is high in carbohydrates and it is metabolised very quickly. It acts like sugar in the body. Some people will be more sensitive to this effect of alcohol than others. You can find out how your glass of wine affects you by keeping a note of how you feel after drinking it. A pattern will emerge. To diminish the effects of alcohol on your blood-sugar levels, make sure that you eat something with your glass of wine. Some people find that their desire for alcohol diminishes if they manage their blood-sugar levels better by not skipping meals and by eating a wholefood diet.

stress

'Stress' is a word we hear a lot about these days. If you pick up any newspaper or magazine, you will probably find an article devoted to this topic and you will most likely read that we are all under a lot of stress. You might think that feeling stressed is a bad thing. But stress is actually an ancient response that is designed to protect us. If we are threatened, we need to be equipped to deal with the threat. The stress response happens in the body when we perceive stress. When we perceive or feel a stressor a number of physiological activities instantly start to take place because the brain believes that there is danger nearby. We need energy, either to confront the danger or to run away from it. This is known as the 'fight or flight' response and this response is how our caveperson ancestor would have reacted when confronted by a tiger. Without it, we would not have the energy to survive encounters with danger.

Stress hormones

Though the stress response really starts in your brain when you become aware of a stressor, the hormones that begin the stress response come from your adrenal glands. Your adrenal glands are two small triangular glands that sit on top of your kidneys. They are endocrine glands, which means that they secrete the hormones they make directly into the bloodstream. The adrenals are also near the liver and the pancreas; organs which are both involved in the stress response and therefore need to have rapid access to adrenal hormones. The major stress hormones influence almost every body function. The adrenal glands produce a variety of hormones: these include adrenaline, which

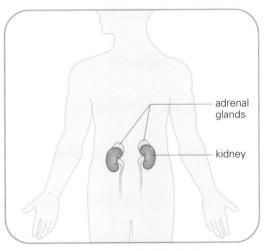

The location of the adrenal glands in the body

adrenal glands

kidney

77

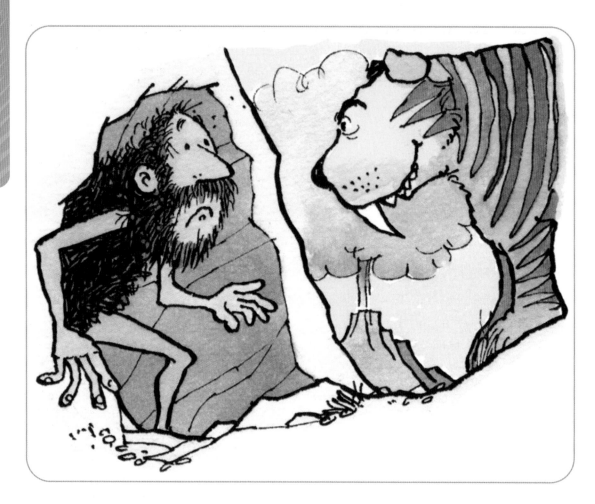

is needed during the very beginning of the stress response; aldosterone, which helps to regulate sodium levels in your body; the sex hormones oestrogen, progesterone and testosterone; and cortisol.

Cortisol

Cortisol is needed for prolonged periods of stress. Life cannot be supported without it. However, when cortisol is produced in excess, as might be the case with an unrelenting, ongoing stress response, this situation can seriously diminish the quality of life. Because of the significance of maintaining a proper level of cortisol in the body, we will focus

on the functions of cortisol, the consequences of inadequate and excessive cortisol levels, what initiates the secretion of cortisol and how appropriate levels of cortisol can be maintained through nutrition and lifestyle practices.

How stress makes us feel

As you read this, take a few minutes to imagine how you feel when you feel very stressed. You might say that you feel anxious, nauseous, teary, angry and shaky, or that your heart beats faster and your breathing is more rapid but shallow. If you are under stress a lot of the time, you might be told that you have high blood pressure.

These feelings aren't very pleasant, but if you think of the stress response in terms of what it was designed for – a caveperson confronting a tiger – you will be able to understand what is happening in your body. Remember that your body still perceives stress in these ancient terms. Let's look at some of these stress-response reactions and think of them in terms of someone confronting danger.

What happens in the body

When you are undergoing the stress response, the following events happen:

- Your heart rate rises. This is to move blood with glucose and oxygen faster to your muscles so that you will have more energy to fight or run from the tiger.

- The blood vessels that supply blood to your skin and the organs that are not needed for fighting constrict, while the blood vessels supplying blood to the lungs, heart, skeletal muscles and brain dilate. The overall constriction leads to higher blood pressure to counteract the possibility of a rapid drop in blood pressure if there is a severe wound as a result of fighting. The digestive and reproductive organs do not receive the energy they normally need because your body assumes that when you are fighting a tiger you are not lying under a bush digesting your meal, nor are you lying under a bush procreating!

- Your liver releases stored carbohydrate into your bloodstream as glucose and your body also starts to make more glucose from your own body proteins because it thinks you will need the extra sugar for energy for fighting. So when you are under stress, your blood-sugar levels rise.

- Cortisol is a natural anti-inflammatory hormone so cortisol levels also rise because your body thinks you might need an anti-inflammatory if you are wounded.

- Your cholesterol levels may also rise because it is the starter material for making cortisol and all the other adrenal hormones.

So when you are stressed, the feelings you have are due to the physiological activities of the stress response.

Modern 'tigers'

We are rarely confronted by real tigers these days, but we may have modern 'tigers' that make your body have the same stress response. These are your stressors. You will be aware of some of your stressors, but there may be others that you may not be aware of. Stressors you know about may be a job that you don't like, a boss that gives you a hard time, a teacher who is very strict, or a relationship that is not a happy one. Stressors you may not be aware of include food sensitivities or allergies, undiagnosed infections, poor blood-sugar control, dehydration, nutrient deficiencies, too much exercise, drugs, exposure to pollution, xeno-oestrogens, toxin exposure, parasites or poor sleep patterns. All of these modern 'tigers' can result in prolonged elevated cortisol levels.

You may have more than one 'tiger' to cope with. For example, you may be a single mother and you have a stressful job you cannot afford to leave. Because you have very little time, you eat refined convenience foods, which elevate your blood-sugar levels. You may have an undiagnosed infection such as a lingering cold or flu virus, be sleeping badly because of stress but also because one of your small children is not sleeping through the night. In the morning, you want caffeine and lots of sugar because you are desperate for energy. In this situation, you have a lot of 'tigers'!

79

The effects of prolonged stress

The stress response is designed to be of short duration. It occurs when the brain perceives a stressor and starts to react. The example we have used is that of a caveperson suddenly being confronted by a tiger. This confrontation is supposed to be over with once the tiger has been killed or the caveperson has successfully escaped. When the situation that caused the stress response is resolved, cortisol levels diminish and the caveperson is then able to get on with activities that occur in a time of relaxation or where there is no perceived threat, such as eating and being able to digest food. The problem with our modern 'tigers' is that they just aren't going away. This changes the picture from one alternating between times of stress and times of relaxation to one where there is just ongoing stress. This results in elevated cortisol levels that are ongoing.

Why are elevated cortisol levels a problem? In Chapter 6 you saw that elevated insulin levels are a problem. You will learn more about the problems of having elevated insulin levels in Chapter 8. The same is true for cortisol. Both are hormones and hormones need to be balanced, with their levels neither too high nor too low. If your cortisol levels are too high over a long period of time, your adrenal glands will become exhausted by the need to produce high levels of cortisol all the time. Eventually, they can become depleted and then it will be difficult for them to produce high levels of cortisol even when they receive messages from

casestudy: Ellie the exercise junkie

Ellie, in her late thirties, came into my office complaining of extreme fatigue. In fact, she spent our entire interview session lying on the couch in my office because she did not have the energy to sit up. I was alarmed when she asked me to dim the bright lights in the office. There were no bright lights. Such sensitivity to light can be a sign of extreme adrenal exhaustion. In taking her case history I was shocked when she told me that only a year before, she had been very athletic and was doing technical rock climbing and regularly entered marathons and triathlons. Later, an adrenal stress test showed that Ellie's adrenals were extremely depleted and this meant that she was having great difficulty in meeting life's daily demands. Ellie was facing some really nasty 'tigers': she was insulin-resistant and probably had been so for a very long time. She had lived on energy bars and power bars as her major source of nutrition during her athletic

pursuits. These are very processed foods and most of them have a high amount of sugar. They are also full of chopped, baked grains. Tests showed that Ellie was gluten-intolerant. She came to realise that a wholefood diet would serve her well. She also knew that she was so fatigued that exercise of any kind was out of the question until she could start to rebuild her depleted adrenal glands. Ellie agreed that she needed rest and good nutrition and set about making sure that her blood-sugar levels got under control. She recovered very slowly as her adrenal glands were so exhausted. After six months of diligent work on her health, she felt 80 per cent better than she had when I first saw her. Ellie realised that she would not be able to return to her previous level of exercise and that the changes she had made were lifestyle changes, but she was quite happy with that since, as she put it, 'I got my life back.'

the brain telling them to do so. If you have reached this stage of adrenal exhaustion, you will be extremely fatigued.

Stress and your hormones

The hormones in your body are always striving for balance. They operate in relation to each other. There is a direct connection between adrenal stress and the thyroid. When chronic stress occurs and the adrenal glands are producing excessive cortisol, the thyroid slows down. Some research has shown that the thyroid slows down in response to adrenal overdrive, because one of the functions of cortisol is the conversion of body proteins to glucose for extra energy. If the body is in a constant breakdown state and is not rebuilding itself, then the thyroid might slow down in order to stop the breakdown of body tissue. Remember, the thyroid is in control of the rate of metabolism in the body. If the

thyroid slows for this reason, then it might show up in a blood test as low thyroid. Sometimes these people don't do well on thyroid medication because the problem really starts with adrenal function. Nutritional therapists have seen people who have been diagnosed with thyroid problems get better when they address their adrenal function and stress levels, as well as their thyroid function.

Stress and the menopause

Before the menopause, oestrogen is mostly produced by the ovaries. After menopause, the ovaries stop producing oestrogen but the adrenal glands take over this production. If you are menopausal, under a lot of stress and your adrenal glands are depleted, producing oestrogen will be a difficult task for your adrenal glands. Stress-management techniques and rebuilding your adrenal glands through good nutrition will be very important for your overall health.

Nutritional help for stress

Here are some dietary and lifestyle suggestions for addressing stress nutritionally. First, use your DAL record (see Chapter 6) to record several days of your eating and activity habits. Try to identify if you have some 'tigers' that you are not aware of, such as poor blood-sugar control, food sensitivities or nutrient deficiencies caused by consuming sugar and refined foods. Also look what you are drinking. Here are some questions to help you:

- Do you notice that you consume a lot of sugar, refined carbohydrates, alcohol or caffeine?

- Do you skip meals?

- Might you be dehydrated?

- Can you identify any patterns of digestive problems after eating certain foods?

If you answered 'Yes' to any of these questions, here are some suggestions for nutritional and lifestyle strategies to help you manage your 'tigers':

- Follow the general guidelines for a healthier diet as outlined in Chapter 1, but avoid any foods you think you might be intolerant to. You might want to 'challenge' these foods. See Chapter 11.

- Follow the guidelines for maximising your digestion given in Chapter 5. Remember that your digestion is impaired if you are under stress because its energy is being diverted to the organs and systems involved in fighting your 'tigers'. While you work on managing your stress levels, take as much work off your digestive system as possible.

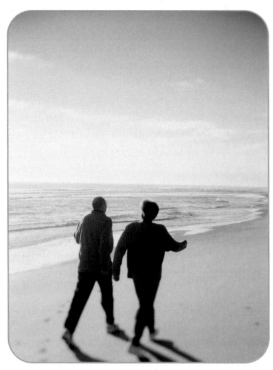

Some exercise helps to reduce stress

❧ Poor blood-sugar control is the second greatest stressor to the body after mental and emotional stress. Pay special attention to managing your blood sugar. See Chapter 6.

❧ Incorporate some stress-management strategies to allow yourself more relaxation time and to give your adrenal glands a chance to rest and rebuild. (See two other books in this series: *Stress Management in Essence* and *Aromatherapy in Essence*.)

❧ If you smoke, please consider giving it up. Smoking drastically depletes the body of nutrients and since it is toxic, it is another 'tiger'.

❧ If you do not exercise regularly, begin a regular exercise programme. However, be careful not to do too much. Exercise can help to alleviate stress, but if you overdo it, it can become a 'tiger' and elevate your

cortisol levels. Walking is a good form of exercise. If you have extreme fatigue, even walking might be too much to begin with. If you need help with designing a fitness programme that is right for you, consult a fitness trainer.

❧ If you are under a lot of stress, you may also crave caffeine. Caffeine artificially boosts your adrenal glands. But caffeine is a double-edged sword; though it makes you feel more energised if you are depleted, in reality it is depleting your body even further. This is a difficult craving to be rid of. Try to cut back on your caffeine intake and, if you can, eliminate it. If this is difficult for you, consult the advice of a nutritional therapist who can help you to cut down.

❧ Ongoing stress rapidly uses vitamin C. Incorporate foods that are high in this vitamin. These include citrus fruits, peppers, broccoli, cantaloupe, strawberries and tomatoes.

❧ Vitamin B5 directly feeds the adrenal glands. However, it is a good idea to take B vitamins together. Incorporate foods that are high in the B vitamins. A wholefood diet will contain all the B vitamins with the exceptions noted for vitamin B12 (see Chapter 3).

❧ Maintaining a good potassium-to-sodium ratio is very beneficial. A wholefood diet will naturally be higher in potassium than sodium, but adding in the Vital Vegetable Broth as a drink (see Chapter 1) will help even more. Try drinking a mug or two of hot broth in the late afternoon, which is when our adrenal glands are normally at their lowest performance level. You might also try it as your first drink of the morning. Vegetables, especially the leafy greens, have a higher potassium-to-sodium ratio.

Zinc and magnesium are minerals that are vulnerable to depletion during times of stress. Incorporate foods that are high in these minerals. Wholegrains, nuts, seeds, leafy green vegetables, shellfish and the dark meat of turkey are examples of these foods. Follow the directions for preparing grains in Chapter 5 to ensure maximum digestion of them.

FAQs

I have a very stressful job and I get ill a lot. I seem to catch every cold and flu virus that's going around. Is there a connection?
There can be. Remember that cortisol levels are only supposed to be elevated for the time that the caveperson is confronted with a tiger. The confrontation is over once the tiger has been dealt with, and cortisol levels diminish. When cortisol is elevated initially, it stimulates your immune system. This can be helpful in fighting infection. However, if your immune system has been stimulated over a long period of time, it becomes exhausted and its efficiency can be challenged. So, in your situation, it's very important to learn ways of managing your stress levels and to optimise your nutrition by following a wholefood diet.

You give examples of how we are exposed to multiple 'tigers' that won't go away. Some of these we cannot just give up, like a job or our family. What are we supposed to do in this situation?
This depends on your situation and also how you manage it. Something that stresses you may not affect someone else as badly. You may have a lot of stressors and on a particularly bad day it may all seem too much. The same difficult day, for someone without other stressors, may not tax them too much. For example, you could have two students about to take the same exam. One student feels ill with the stress associated with taking the exam, while the other is relaxed. This gives a clue about stress management. All of your modern 'tigers' are like layers of an onion. If you can peel away some of them, the others might not seem as severe as they did before. Even though you can't give up your job or leave your family, you can balance your blood sugar better and avoid eating foods you are sensitive to. My experience with clients who do this is that after a few weeks their job and family 'tigers' become more like tiger cubs.

83

weight loss

Diet and nutrition myth: *Weight loss is simple. It's all about 'calories in, calories out'. So if you eat less and exercise more, you will always automatically lose weight.*

Weight loss is one of the main reasons people seek out the help of a nutritional therapist. Many of us try diet after diet: we lose some weight, then put it straight back on again when we come off the diet. Some diets advocate the consumption of lots of one particular food for days on end that is 'guaranteed to melt off the pounds'. Or we may copy a friend who found a particular weight-loss programme very successful, only to find that when we try it, it doesn't work for us. Added to the frustration of dieting is the fact that many of the so-called 'experts' out there are still telling us that weight loss is simply a matter of 'calories in, calories out'. They tell us that if we exercise more and eat less, we would lose the weight easily. But for many of us, this doesn't work.

If you have tried unsuccessfully to lose weight, you will find this chapter interesting. Blood sugar (Chapter 6), stress (Chapter 7) and the immune system (Chapter 11) as well as digestion and detoxification (Chapter 5) can also affect weight loss.

How much food should we eat?

Portion control is important. Many of us have little idea of the amount of food our bodies really need. You may think it is best to severely restrict the amount of calories you eat. However, it's very important not to skip meals. This may seem like odd advice if you still believe that weight loss is just a matter of cutting calories and it's a good thing to miss meals during a busy day. However, if you don't eat until the evening, it makes it very difficult not to overeat when you do allow your body some food. Your body needs regular intakes of the right foods.

The number of calories you are taking in obviously does matter, but counting calories is not the whole story to weight loss. How your body processes the food you give it plays as big a role in weight management as how much you eat.

The ideal meal

Rather than measuring out and counting calories, the best way to estimate the correct amounts of food you need is to divide up your plate. The following example shows a plate for a meal that contains good proportions of the right kind of foods.

Most of the plate has a variety of low-carbohydrate vegetables such as leafy greens and green beans. A smaller portion of the plate has high-carbohydrate vegetables such as potatoes. A quarter of the plate has protein and fat sources such as fatty fish, hard-boiled eggs, olives, avocado and the dressing, which could be a mixture of olive oil and lemon juice.

Alternatively, you could have a meal where you steamed some vegetables and then drizzled about a tablespoon of coconut oil over the vegetables. Or you might have most of your plate filled with a mixed stir-fry which has these same proportions of vegetables, proteins and fats; or you could have a bowl of soup or stew that has the same proportions of

these foods. This gives you a rough idea of how to gauge portions. Low-carbohydrate vegetables are very low in calories. If you follow these examples and you are eating wholefoods, the calories will automatically take care of themselves.

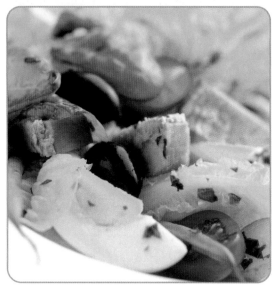

A salad niçoise

Cravings

One of the commonest problems with diets and food deprivation is cravings. Cravings are usually associated with low blood-sugar levels, caused by eating sugar or refined carbohydrates, skipping meals, a lack of protein and good fats in the diet and sometimes an overgrowth in the intestines of the yeast candida. (You can read more about these issues in other chapters in this book.) Cravings are not your fault! They occur for these reasons, not because you don't have willpower. If your blood-sugar levels drop too low, your brain is not being fed the glucose it needs. Your brain will not allow itself to starve. It will do anything to correct this situation, and this includes sending you some very powerful signals that

you need to eat. When the brain needs glucose, it sends you signals to eat sugar, so that it gets glucose very quickly. The solution is to avoid letting your brain get low on glucose. This is why skipping meals is not a good idea.

How the good fats can help

Cravings for sugar can be alleviated by ensuring that you have some of the good fats in your diet. It is sugar that makes you gain weight, not necessarily fats! But the fats you eat need to be good fats, such as olive oil or from nuts and seeds. The bad fats, such as the hydrogenated fats and trans fats, can make you gain weight because they are toxic to your system. Good fats can actually make you more metabolically active, which means that you will burn more calories if you eat them. (Refer to Chapter 2 for a discussion on fats.) The problem with sugar is that it raises insulin levels. Insulin is necessary for life, but in excess, it can be damaging. Insulin is a fat-sparing hormone, which means that if you have high levels of insulin in your blood, signals are sent within your body to store and conserve fat, not burn it. Therefore you could be running on a treadmill all day long to try to burn fat, but it won't happen because your body is getting chemical messages from the high levels of insulin in your blood to hang onto that fat! Now you can begin to see how weight loss is not simply a matter of 'calories in, calories out'. The secret is to keep your blood-sugar levels stable. You can do this by eating regular meals that include healthy fats and protein. But keep an eye on the amounts – remember the 'ideal meal' described earlier.

Stress and weight gain

Stress makes you fat. Chapter 7 outlines how constant stress results in elevated levels of cortisol. Remember that cortisol is not a 'bad' hormone: in fact, you cannot live without it. However, as with insulin, chronically elevated levels of cortisol are not good for your health. The key is to strive for balance. Remember that your body is designed to function as bodies did during the time of our ancestors. Back then, there were times of feast and times of famine. There were times when people were faced with a sudden tiger and peaceful times when they could lie happily under a bush digesting their food. The answer here is to manage your stress levels so that you do not feel stressed all the time.

When you are stressed and your stressors or 'modern tigers' aren't going away, cortisol is elevated. This is because the body is gearing up for a fight. To fight, you need energy. One of the things cortisol does is to encourage your body to make energy from sources other than carbohydrates such as protein. This means that it has the ability to tell your body to start breaking down your own body proteins (such as your muscles) to make sugar which then enters the blood. High levels of sugar in the blood cause insulin to be produced, but this elevated cortisol situation also encourages insulin. So you can have a situation where you have high blood-sugar levels, high insulin levels in the blood and high cortisol. This situation encourages weight gain which is particularly noticeable around the abdominal area.

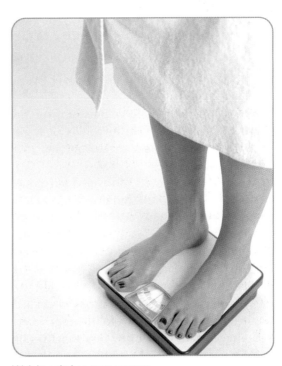

Weight gain has many causes

casestudy: Andrea's abdomen

Andrea, a 40-year-old client, was very concerned about what she thought was recent weight gain. She told me that her clothes were getting tighter and tighter and she wanted a programme that would help her to lose weight. Her DAL records (see Chapter 6) looked OK: her portion control was good, she was getting regular exercise and she was eating mostly wholefoods. Furthermore, she did not look overweight to me at all. She actually had quite thin arms and legs. Her weight gain was a mystery until I asked her if she was weighing herself and where on her body she felt she was gaining weight. She was not weighing herself, but she felt her abdomen getting bigger, She had had to buy a larger size of jeans. It turned out that Andrea had not gained weight. She had a bloated abdomen due to her ongoing stress levels and insulin resistance. She started a stress-management programme and worked hard at balancing her blood-sugar levels. Within a couple of months, her abdomen was much flatter and she felt much more comfortable.

You can also have abdominal swelling if you eat foods to which you are sensitive. (Chapter 11 has more information on this.) An intolerance to gluten (the sticky protein found in wheat and certain other grains) is the most common food intolerance. People in the Hollywood movie industry know this secret well: years ago a well-known actress in her forties was asked how she was able to keep her stomach so flat. She replied: 'I don't eat wheat!' Ongoing inflammation in the intestines due to a food intolerance causes swelling. It is also a stressful condition for the body and elevates cortisol levels. Another reason why weight gain is not simply about 'calories in, calories out'.

Dieting and your thyroid

A history of past dieting can also impair the action of the thyroid. Your thyroid is the organ of the endocrine system that maintains your metabolic rate.

If you have low levels of thyroid hormones (hypothyroid), you will find it difficult to lose weight because your metabolism will be abnormally slow. This is a medical condition and you can have your thyroid checked by your doctor.

There are two nutritional connections to low thyroid. One is a past history of cyclical dieting (also known as 'yo-yo' dieting) where you are deprived of calories, lose weight, gain it back, diet, lose weight, gain it back and so

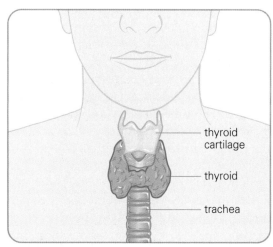

thyroid cartilage

thyroid

trachea

The thyroid

on. Over time, your thyroid decides that you are in a period of starvation and lowers its activity, causing you to conserve energy.

The other nutritional condition that causes thyroid problems involves the immune system. Sometimes there is a connection between gluten intolerance and an autoimmune condition where your immune system attacks your thyroid, thinking it is a pathogen because it does not recognise it as part of your body. This is another important reason to identify any food sensitivities you may have. In addition to asking your doctor to test your thyroid, you can ask to be tested for thyroid antibodies. If you have a positive result to thyroid antibodies, you might try avoiding gluten (found in wheat and most other grains) and any other foods to which you are intolerant, then get your thyroid tested again after two or three months to see if the results are different. (See Chapter 11 for more about gluten.)

In a nutshell recipe:

Cauliflower instead of potatoes

Potatoes are very nutritious, especially if you eat the skins. But they are very starchy and can have an effect in raising blood-sugar levels if eaten alone. Cauliflower can be used as a substitute for potatoes, in many cases. For example, try steaming or boiling some cauliflower and then mashing it.

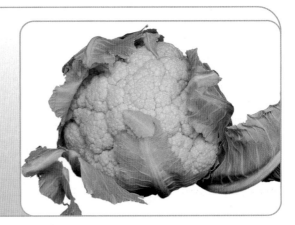

Nutritional help for weight loss

Here are some dietary and lifestyle suggestions for weight loss:

First, use your DAL record (see Chapter 6) to record several days of your eating and activity habits. Here are some questions to help you:

- Are you eating appropriate portions at every meal?
- Are you skipping meals?
- Do you get regular exercise?
- Do you notice any times when you feel bloated or have abdominal swelling? If so, can you associate these times with eating a particular food?

Once you have a sense of your eating patterns, here are some suggestions you might incorporate for a healthy weight-loss plan:

- Follow the general guidelines for a healthier diet.
- Don't skip meals. Keep your blood-sugar levels stable.
- Eat small amounts of protein at every meal.

- ⚘ If you don't get any exercise, consider a regular exercise program. Walking is a good way to start.

- ⚘ If you are under a lot of stress, consider following a stress-management programme.

- ⚘ Try to get good, sustained sleep every night. There is an association with chronic sleep deprivation and weight gain.

- ⚘ If you smoke, give it up. Once you do, your body will balance itself after being off cigarettes for a while.

- ⚘ Look at what you are drinking. If you drink soft drinks or alcohol, they are adding sugar to your diet. If you regularly visit a coffee shop and typically order a latte frappuchino deluxe, consider inquiring how many calories there are in those drinks. You might be shocked.

- ⚘ Use healthy fats such as organic butter, ghee, coconut oil or olive oil for cooking and don't consume margarine, hydrogenated fats or trans fats.

- ⚘ Include wild, cold-water fatty fish, or flax seeds, walnuts and leafy greens in your diet to ensure you get the Omega-3 fats in your diet. Lightly grind the flax seeds in a spice or coffee grinder just before you use them.

- ⚘ Choose most of your carbohydrates from vegetables, especially the low-carbohydrate ones.

In a nutshell recipe:

Basic vinaigrette

Many bottled salad dressings contain cheap processed oils that are not healthy choices. You can make a simple and quick vinaigrette of your own. A classic vinaigrette salad dressing consists of a ratio of one part acid to three or four parts fat. The acid usually consists of vinegar, but you can also use lemon juice. The fat is usually an extra-virgin olive oil. For a lighter-tasting version, try using rice vinegar as your vinegar source.

Acid and oil don't normally blend well. To enhance the blending, put your acid and any herbs or seasonings into a glass salad-dressing bottle (with a lid) first and then add in the oil little by little, shaking the bottle well after each addition. This kind of dressing will keep for about a week in the refrigerator. You can add flavourings such as sea salt, cracked pepper, fresh or dried herbs or a little mustard. You might even try adding a teaspoon of the Powerfull Pesto recipe in Chapter 5.

FAQs

How can I follow a weight-loss plan and still go out to eat at restaurants?

Eating out can be a challenge. Remember portions! Choose oily fish or lean meats, and vegetables that don't have creamy or cheese sauces on them. If you order a salad, ask for vinaigrette and ask to have the dressing on the side. Dip your fork in the dressing before picking up a bite of salad. Avoid the bread basket if you can!

What are some good snack ideas for a working person on a weight-loss plan?

Assuming that you can eat these foods and don't have a food sensitivity to them, you could try:

- an apple and a small piece of cheese
- apple slices with almond butter
- one hard-boiled egg with tomato slices
- prewashed, organic greens from the supermarket (to make it more interesting, you could add in a small amount of raw nuts and seeds)
- an oatcake with nut butter.

I love some crunch in my salad but I don't want to eat croutons on my weight-loss plan. What can I do?

Replace the croutons with some slivered lightly roasted almonds. (Note: Though nuts and seeds are recommended, make sure you watch the total amount you eat in a day – too many can add up the calories.)

I work and am trying to lose weight. At work I often don't have time to eat and I often replace meals with drinks, such as lattes. I do get exercise after work, but I still find that I cannot lose any weight. What's my problem?

One consideration might be what you are drinking. Many people believe that liquids are low in calories but this can be a false belief. Add up the calories of your lattes and the other drinks you are drinking and you might be surprised! Try replacing them with herb teas, water and Vital Vegetable Broth (Chapter 1).

women's health

This chapter looks at how nutrition affects women's health. After fatigue, the main reason women seek the advice of a nutritional therapist is because they believe their female hormones may be out of balance. The main female hormones are oestrogen and progesterone (though men have these hormones as well, in lesser amounts). A woman's hormone levels are individual to her and there are many fluctuations and differing levels from woman to woman. Symptoms of an imbalance in these hormones include premenstrual syndrome (PMS), adverse symptoms associated with menopause, polycystic ovarian syndrome (PCOS), depression or migraines associated with a woman's cycle and infertility.

Sometimes the real reason behind an imbalance in female hormones is not a problem with the hormones themselves. Many of the conditions seen as female hormone conditions can be alleviated by the same dietary strategies used to balance blood sugar (Chapter 6), employing better stress management if you are stressed due to the adrenal / blood-sugar connection (Chapter 7), paying attention to the fats in your diet and bringing in the good fats and avoiding the bad fats (Chapter 2) to reduce inflammation, and considering if you should try a dietary programme in detoxification since it is the job of your liver to break down old oestrogen and also to detoxify xeno-oestrogens (Chapter 5). If you are a woman who has hormonal issues, a new approach towards balancing your hormones is to consider yourself a person first and then a woman. If you address your nutritional issues, you might find that your hormonal symptoms are alleviated or that they even disappear.

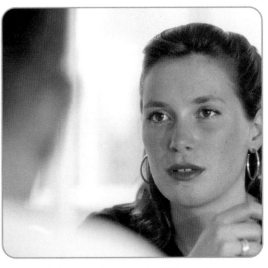
A woman's hormone levels are individual to her

93

If you are under medical care, check with your doctor to determine how best to use these nutritional strategies along with any medication you are taking. You might also ask to get your thyroid checked if you think you may have a low thyroid (See Chapter 8).

How female hormones work

In a standard 'textbook' example, from the end of a woman's period until she ovulates, there is a rise in her level of oestrogen. Oestrogen encourages cell growth by building up the endometrium. It also nourishes the endometrium by increasing blood supply to it so that the woman's womb is ready for one of her eggs to be implanted if that egg is fertilised. Ovulation occurs, and in 'textbook woman' this is two weeks from the end of her last menses. (In real-life women, this time period can vary). For the next two weeks before a woman's next period begins, progesterone levels rise and become greater than oestrogen levels. Progesterone ripens the endometrium in case fertilisation occurs and an egg needs to be implanted. If fertilisation does not occur, then oestrogen and progesterone levels fall and the endometrium is shed from the uterus, resulting in the next period. In reality, however, women's cycles vary. If a cycle is too long or too short, or if oestrogen and progesterone do not rise and fall in the described pattern, the woman may be told that her hormones are out of balance.

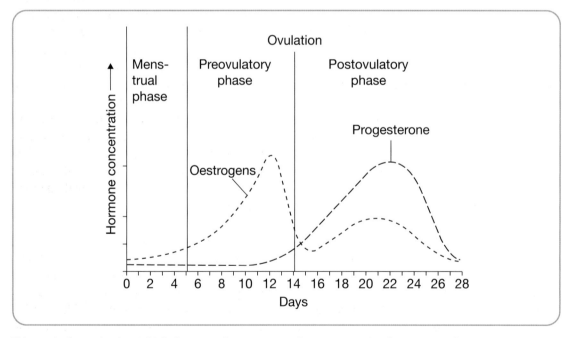

This graph shows the rise and fall of a woman's oestrogen and progesterone levels over a month

Hormone health problems

Let's look at some of the female health problems normally associated with an imbalance of hormones.

Oestrogen dominance

You may remember from Chapter 5 that the liver breaks down and regulates hormones such as oestrogen. If old oestrogen is not clearing from the body adequately, the body will have elevated levels of oestrogen in relation to progesterone. This will also be the case if there is exposure to xeno-oestrogens – the harmful 'false oestrogen' chemical substances. Xeno-oestrogens are converted in the liver to a form of oestrogen known as '16-OH', which is carcinogenic. If you have a higher amount of oestrogen compared to your progesterone, you are in oestrogen dominance.

As we have seen, hormones work best if they are in balance with each other. Elevated cortisol or insulin levels can also lead to oestrogen dominance. Oestrogen dominance can play a role in PMS, PCOS, the development of fibroids, endometriosis and breast cancer. If you think you are oestrogen-dominant, using nutritional strategies targeted towards balancing all the hormones in your body and undergoing a nutritional liver support programme might be a good idea.

Oestrogen in menopause

Even if you are a woman in menopause and have low oestrogen levels, you can still be in oestrogen dominance if your progesterone levels are also low, so that the ratio of oestrogen to progesterone is still higher. The balance exists in the ratio between the two hormones. This is one reason some researchers now believe that there is a link between the use of HRT in menopause and cancer: even though a woman's oestrogen levels are low, if her progesterone is also low and she is in oestrogen dominance, giving her additional oestrogen could put her at risk of developing breast cancer.

Progesterone cream

Some health practitioners advocate giving a woman who has oestrogen dominance additional progesterone to counteract her excess oestrogen. This hormone may be administered as a cream that is absorbed through the skin. Any woman who is taking progesterone cream should be tested for her hormone levels. This is because the ability to absorb this hormone differs from woman to woman. Testing has shown that even though a group of women were using the same amount of cream every day, some had absorbed little of it and their progesterone levels were still low, while other women had easily absorbed the cream, and after repeated use there was a build-up of progesterone so that the levels had shot up. Remember, hormones need to be in balance with each other and if one is wildly out of balance, it can adversely affect the balance of hormones in all body systems. Therefore there can be problems associated with elevated levels of progesterone, as well as with elevated oestrogen.

Hormone testing

A healthcare practitioner and a nutritional therapist well-versed in these issues can order testing for you so that you can determine how well your hormones are balanced. This kind of testing can also monitor how you respond to any kind of hormonal therapy rather than assuming that you and all other women will respond in the same uniform, predictable way that a 'textbook' woman would.

women's health

95

Premenstrual syndrome (PMS)

PMS occurs around the beginning of a woman's period. Some women experience symtoms for a week or more before their period starts. Symptoms vary, but include bloating, water retention and weight gain, moodiness, cramps, headaches and breast tenderness. Some women have cravings as well, especially for sugar or chocolate.

It is so common in the UK to have symptoms that most women think that feeling unwell is naturally associated with having a period. However, the symptoms of PMS can be reduced or avoided altogether. In some parts of the world, women do not report experiencing PMS. Nutritional deficiencies such as of magnesium, zinc and B-vitamins can play a role. Blood-sugar imbalances, stress, a lack of good fats and the inclusion of hydrogenated and trans fats in your diet can also make PMS worse, as can exposure to toxicity. If you experience PMS, it is worth looking at your diet and how to manage stress.

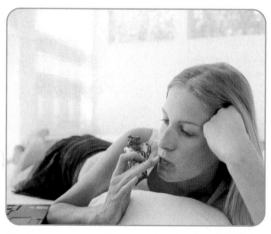
Some women crave chocolate when they have PMS

Polycystic ovarian syndrome (PCOS)

This is a syndrome in which there are cysts on the ovaries. Obesity, elevated insulin, elevated blood sugar and poor blood-fat management can also be present if you have this condition. You may remember seeing many of these problems listed in Chapter 6, about blood sugar. PCOS is strongly linked with insulin resistance. Managing blood-sugar levels is very important for women who face this problem.

Endometriosis and fibroids

Endometriosis is a condition in which the tissue from the endometrium migrates out of the uterus and into other parts of the body. This tissue is as metabolically active as the endometrium so, every month, a woman with endometriosis feels the effect of having her period in various parts of her body. The symptoms usually associated with this condition include severe period pain and backache.

Fibroids are non-cancerous tumours of the uterus. They can cause symptoms such as heavy bleeding and sometimes pain. Both endometriosis and fibroids are thought to be connected to oestrogen dominance.

Menopausal symptoms

Menopause is a natural change when a woman's periods stop. In many societies of the world, the menopause is traditionally celebrated as a time of freedom from menstruation and a time when a woman becomes the 'wise woman' in her society. However, in the West, the time leading up to the menopause – known as perimenopause

– is often associated with negative symptoms. Some women (but by no means all) experience unpleasant symptoms (including hot flushes, dryness of the skin and vagina, insomnia, moodiness and forgetfulness). Some women are even experiencing menopause earlier than their grandmothers did. It is considered to be 'normal' if menopause occurs somewhere between the ages of 45 and 55. It is considered to be premature if it occurs before the age of 40. Poor nutrition or malnourishment,

exposure to toxicity and extreme stress are three reasons why some women are experiencing an earlier menopause than their grandmothers did. Menopause can also be medically induced through various drugs and hysterectomy.

Once a woman's ovaries no longer produce oestrogen, her adrenal glands take over and produce more. So adrenal health is an important consideration in menopause. Good nutrition is especially important.

casestudy: Menopausal Marian

Marian was a client in her early 40s who came for a nutritional consultation complaining of extreme fatigue, hot flushes, dryness and forgetfulness. Her period had been erratic for some time and at the time of the consultation she had not had a period for three months. She was a single mother, under a lot of stress and ran her own business. Her diet consisted primarily of refined processed packaged foods because she felt she had no time to cook or even to eat properly. She often skipped meals and drank coffee instead. Marian was also on a very low-fat diet because she believed that

eating any fat would make her fat. She did not take any exercise. Because she was not feeling well and her energy levels were low, Marian agreed to work on bringing wholefoods into her diet. After six weeks of eating wholefoods, balancing her blood sugar, undergoing a stress-management programme, bringing healthy fats into her diet and avoiding refined foods, sugar and caffeine, Marian was pleased to note that her menopausal symptoms had disappeared. She was also surprised by the return of her periods. Her body was not really ready to go through menopause.

Osteoporosis

You may think of your bones as rigid, unchanging structures but in reality they are constantly being renewed by being built up and broken down by your body. This remodelling is very much governed by different hormones in your body, including the female hormones as well as thyroid and parathyroid hormones. When a woman goes into menopause and her oestrogen levels drop, she is more at risk of losing bone mass. Bones need calcium, magnesium, phosphorus and

manganese. Smoking, caffeine, excessive alcohol, sugar and refined foods accelerate bone loss.

Phosphorous and calcium

Though phosphorus is contained within bone tissue, an excess dietary intake of phosphoric acid can leach calcium from bones. The phosphoric acid content of soft drinks is quite high and regular and excessive consumption of these drinks can be a contributing factor in encouraging the loss of calcium from your bones. Regular exercise, a wholefood diet and a good balance between calcium and magnesium encourage calcium retention. Many women are led to believe that losing calcium from bone means that they need to supplement with more calcium. In reality, our diets contain more calcium than the diets of indigenous Bantu Africans, yet they have little or no osteoporosis. Maintaining a good bone mass is more dependent on discouraging calcium loss from and encouraging calcium retention in bones. If you are in 'calcium loss from bone mode', just adding in more calcium will not be too helpful. Good dietary and lifestyle approaches will help reverse this process.

Depression and anxiety

Depression and anxiety are not unique to women, nor are they only associated with an imbalance of female hormones. However, they can accompany an imbalance of these hormones. Identifying any potential food sensitivities and avoiding those foods, balancing blood sugar and addressing any nutritional deficiencies will often have a positive effect on depression and anxiety. Read the case study given in Chapter 11 to learn how one woman's food sensitivity was linked to her anxiety attacks. When she avoided this food her anxiety disappeared. Of course, nutritional issues are not always the cause of anxiety, but good nutrition can help.

Infertility

Infertility is a medical issue and can be affected by many factors. However, there are some nutritional considerations that should not be neglected if a woman is trying to conceive. The most obvious of these is nutritional deficiencies. If a woman has been on a strict diet or has lost a lot of weight to the point where she is not having periods, it is unlikely that she will be able to support the growth of a baby. Therefore it is important for a woman to ensure that she is eating a nutritious diet if she wants to conceive. Ensuring that the good fats are included in the diet is very important. (See Chapter 2, on fats.)

Nutritional help for balancing hormones

Here are some dietary and lifestyle suggestions for balancing female sex hormones:

✑ Look back through earlier chapters and see if you can identify possible hormonal issues that you might have in addition to any issues with your sex hormones. In particular, look out for any food sensitivities, elevated stress levels or a blood-sugar imbalance. Then you can begin to address these issues nutritionally, if you have not already done so.

✑ Read Chapter 5 again and follow the recommendations for nutritional support for the liver.

You can also incorporate nutritional strategies aimed at better hormone balance:

✑ Follow the general guidelines for a healthier diet as outlined in Chapter 1. Work towards including organic foods and lowering your intake of foods that might have pesticides on them.

- Some health writers advise against consuming animal products such as meat and dairy. They cite that animal produce causes inflammation because of the make-up of the fats in these products. However, this only applies to those products that are not organic, where the animals have been raised on factory farms and have been given growth hormones, antibiotics and grain-based feed which provides an abundance of Omega-6 fats. Meat and unpasteurised dairy that come from animals raised on organic pastures can provide very beneficial fats and nutrients that are supportive of hormonal balance. The essential fat content in these animals is vastly different from that of animals that have been factory-farmed.

- Pay special attention to the fats in your diet, making sure that you include foods with Omega-3 fatty acids and avoid hydrogenated and trans fats. You can also try including the wholefood helper evening primrose oil (EPO), which is high in Gamma-linoleic acid (GLA). GLA is anti-inflammatory. Borage oil, also known as starflower oil, is higher in GLA than EPO, but it has been noted that women seem to do better on EPO.

- Cruciferous vegetables such as broccoli, cauliflower, cabbage, Brussels sprouts and kale contain a substance which, when mixed with stomach acid, form another substance called diindolymethane (DIM). DIM blocks the production of harmful 16-OH oestrogen and encourages the production of good 2-OH oestrogen. If these foods are raw, they are goitrogens and can lower thyroid activity. However, when they are cooked, the amount of DIM is reduced. Lightly steam these foods.

- Lower your intake of alcohol and stimulants such as caffeine. Alcohol is associated with increased levels of oestrogen. Stimulants are irritating to the adrenal glands.

- Be wary of the argument that soya is good for balancing hormones. Read the discussion in Chapter 2 on how much soya to eat and in what forms. Soya can only be beneficial to health if you are not intolerant of it and if it is not eaten in a highly refined form, or in excess.

- You might try including the wholefood helper cod liver oil (which contains vitamins A and D), especially in the winter months when there is little sun and your body is less able to make its own vitamin D. Vitamin A is necessary for reproduction and vitamin D is supportive of oestrogen production and supports maintaining bone mass.

- Nutrient deficiencies that are typically found alongside female hormone issues are the B-vitamins, magnesium, zinc and the essential fatty acids. Not surprisingly, these are the nutrients that are stripped and lost through the refining of foods. Be sure to include foods that are good sources of these nutrients. They are more readily available in a varied wholefood diet.

- Make sure you have fibre in your diet. See Chapter 4 for a discussion on fibre. Fibre helps to remove toxicity from the body.

In a nutshell recipe:

Simple Salmon Teriyaki

This easy salmon recipe provides Omega-3 fats, which are beneficial for women's health. Be sure that the salmon is wild, not farmed, and consult healthfood stores for good-quality sources of soya sauce and mirin. Store-bought bottles of teriyaki sauce often contain preservatives. A traditional Japanese recipe calls for sugar. This can be omitted by increasing the amount of the mirin (a sweet rice wine).

'Teriyaki' means 'glazed and grilled'. You can also use the sauce for chicken.

Serves 4:
4 small wild salmon fillets, bones removed
3 tbsp of mirin
2 tbsp of soya sauce
1 tbsp sesame oil

1 Mix together the mirin and the soya sauce. Pour into a dish and marinade the fillets for an hour, turning them over once.

2 Heat the oil in a frying pan, but not to the point where the oil smokes.

3 Remove the fillets from the marinade and place in the hot pan. Sear the fish on both sides.

4 Add the marinade and cook until the marinade has thickened into a glaze and the fish is cooked through, but not overdone. Be very careful not to burn the sauce as it cooks or it will turn bitter.

5 Serve warm, with any remaining glaze poured over the top. Serve with vegetables.

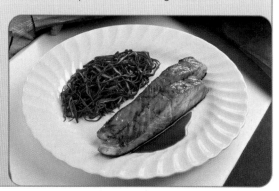

FAQs

I've been told that women should take supplemental iron if we still have periods, because of the blood loss. Is this true?

It is only true if you are anaemic and your doctor has tested you for this. Iron in excess causes oxidation and the formation of harmful free radicals in the body. However, in a woman who is anaemic, it is necessary, so do get your iron levels checked by your doctor. (The levels of iron you take in from wholefoods should not cause a problem.)

Is there a special monthly diet that I should follow to avoid the symptoms of PMS?

The best diet is the healthy diet advocated throughout this book. You should follow it all the time, not just before your period. Managing blood-sugar levels, eating organic wholefoods and ensuring that you include the healthy fats and avoid the bad fats, sugar and refined foods will be your best overall strategy.

Are there nutritional strategies to follow if a woman in on the Pill or HRT?

These are powerful, hormonal drugs and may disrupt hormonal balance. They may also deplete the body of zinc, so eating foods with zinc can be helpful (see Chapter 3 for a list of these foods). Depending on what type of HRT is used, there may be a tendency to produce more of the harmful 16-OH oestrogen. Add foods such as cruciferous vegetables to your diet to produce DIM to help to counteract this. (See 'Nutritional help for balancing hormones', page 98.)

What should I eat to encourage conception?

Following the general guidelines for a healthy diet outlined in this book is your best strategy. Pay special attention to managing your blood-sugar levels and ensure that you include the healthy fats in your diet.

cardiovascular health

Heart disease was not common at the turn of the twentieth century, yet it is now widespread. In this chapter you will learn about some of the nutritional strategies you can follow to have better heart health.

One of the best ways to keep your heart healthy is to get regular exercise. Regular aerobic exercise helps to keep the heart muscle strong. A healthy diet is also critical for maintaining the health of your heart. Some of the information presented in this chapter may differ from traditional nutritional advice you may have seen.

The cardiovascular system

Your heart is part of your cardiovascular system, which also includes your arteries, veins and other smaller blood vessels.

We often discuss heart health, but the health of your blood vessels is critical as well. The umbrella term for diseases that affect the heart or the blood vessels is cardiovascular disease.

The arteries

Your arteries are the large blood vessels that carry blood away from the heart to the tissues. They do the high-pressure work in the body and therefore need to be elastic, flexible and strong. Artery walls are made of smooth muscle and connective tissue and it is this that

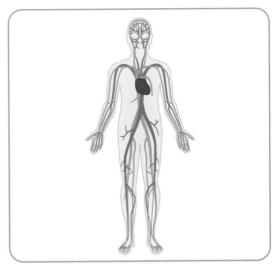

The cardiovascular system – the blue lines are the veins and the red the arteries

103

gives them their strength and flexibility. A lot of activity takes place in the lining of arteries: it can constrict or dilate and release chemicals.

It has been said that you are as old as the health of your arteries. If the condition of the arteries is poor, disorders such as atherosclerosis and hypertension (or high blood pressure) can develop.

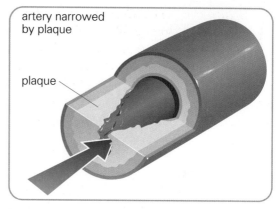

The inside of an artery segment with a plaque build-up

Heart health

Let's discuss some of the problems associated with heart health.

Atherosclerosis

Atherosclerosis is the form of hardening of the arteries where cholesterol, fats and calcium are deposited in the artery walls. If they are not stopped or removed, these deposits can become hard plaques that may block your arteries and lead to a heart attack or stroke.

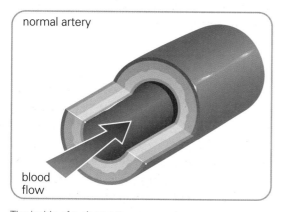

The inside of a clean artery segment

Cholesterol

Many people assume that cholesterol is the 'bad guy' in atherosclerosis and that reducing dietary cholesterol is necessary to reduce the build-up of plaque in the arterial walls. Some people avoid eating animal foods because they contain cholesterol. Yet your liver has the ability to make the body's own cholesterol. Let's look at why this is the case.

- Cholesterol is the starting material for all of your steroid hormones. These include oestrogen, progesterone, testosterone and the stress hormone cortisol, which is made by the adrenal glands. If you have prolonged stress, your liver might make more cholesterol so that you can make more cortisol. If someone has an infection and they need the anti-inflammatory properties of cortisol, their blood-cholesterol levels rise.

- Communication between cells in the body happens on the cell membrane. Cell membranes need to have the right amount of stiffness and the right amount of fluidity to function well. Cholesterol provides the rigidity factor that each cell membrane needs.

🖎 Higher levels of cholesterol are found in brain tissue. Breast milk has high levels of cholesterol in it. Research shows that cholesterol appears to play an important role in the brain development of babies.

So, while it is true that you would not want your arteries blocked with cholesterol, it does have its uses in the body.

Cholesterol questions

1 'If your liver makes cholesterol, does the cholesterol you eat really make a difference in your blood levels of cholesterol?' Studies have shown that the answer is: 'No, not if the cholesterol is from wholefoods.' Except for a very small percentage of people, dietary cholesterol from foods does not have an effect on blood-cholesterol levels, unless the food contains oxidised and damaged cholesterol.

2 'Why does cholesterol block arteries?' Oxidised and damaged cholesterol is found in processed foods that have been heated to high temperatures, such as powdered eggs and milk. So the answer is: 'The kind of cholesterol that blocks arteries is typically oxidised or damaged cholesterol.'

The idea that cholesterol in the diet is not a cause of heart disease makes sense if you consider that there are indigenous people such as the Inuit (Eskimos) who live on a diet that is very high in cholesterol, yet their level of cardiovascular disease is low.

Lipoproteins

The other substance in blood tests that is often labelled 'bad' is low-density lipoprotein (LDL). It is often referred to as the 'bad cholesterol'. Its counterpart, HDL, or high-density lipoprotein, is called the 'good cholesterol'. Doctors sometimes tell patients that they want to see their levels of 'bad' cholesterol lowered, and higher levels of their 'good' cholesterol.

LDL and HDL are not only cholesterol. They are lipoproteins (substances that are proteins bound with fats). They act as carriers in the blood. Blood is watery and it is the transport medium throughout the body. Fat and water don't mix, so if fatty substances need to be transported via the blood, they need to be escorted by other substances that are more soluble.

Many doctors are now looking at the ratio of HDL and LDL levels. Even if a person's total cholesterol level is high and their LDL level is high, if the HDL level is high enough (especially in relation to their LDL level), then they are likely to be considered at low risk of cardiovascular disease.

Triglycerides

Another cardiovascular marker that is measured in conventional medicine is your level of triglycerides. Triglycerides are building blocks of lipoproteins. Often, irrespective of total cholesterol levels, low HDL levels and high triglyceride levels are related to eating too many carbohydrates in your diet. This is especially true if the carbohydrates are refined.

Inflammation

Some researchers are beginning to look at inflammation as a marker of cardiovascular disease (rather than just focusing on cholesterol). Where inflammation occurs, it is like the body being on fire in that area. If you get a cut on your finger it becomes inflamed: there is heat, redness and pain. In this case, the inflammation is a sign of your immune system protecting you. It speeds up reactions and brings nutrients and immune cells to the wound more quickly, so that pathogens can be killed. As soon as your immune system has handled the invading pathogens, the inflammation subsides. However, the kind of unrelenting inflammation that causes heart disease is not beneficial to the body.

Homocysteine

Blood tests can be used to measure inflammation. One such test measures homocysteine levels. Homocysteine is a substance that is like an amino acid and is a by-product of protein metabolism. It is normal to have some homocysteine in your blood, as it is an intermediate product in the process where the amino acid methionine is being made into the amino acid cysteine. However, this conversion is dependent on the presence of three vitamins: vitamin B12, vitamin B6 and folic acid. If there is a deficiency in these vitamins, homocysteine can build up and levels of it can rise in your blood.

A small number of people have a genetic problem with homocysteine build-up. Homocysteine is a cause of cardiovascular disease because it is a highly inflammatory substance which creates free radicals and causes the formation of the cholesterol plaques in the arteries. This irritating substance can cause nicks and scratches in the arteries, which isn't good news as arteries do the high-pressure work in the body.

Quenching inflammation

It is often thought that it is cholesterol that is blocking the artery when it arrives there with LDL. But if we think of inflammation as the body on fire, cholesterol is the firefighter and LDL is the fire engine. If you undertake strategies to lower cholesterol and LDL and do nothing about homocysteine and issues causing inflammation, you are allowing the fire to burn and you are making the firefighters and their fire engines leave the

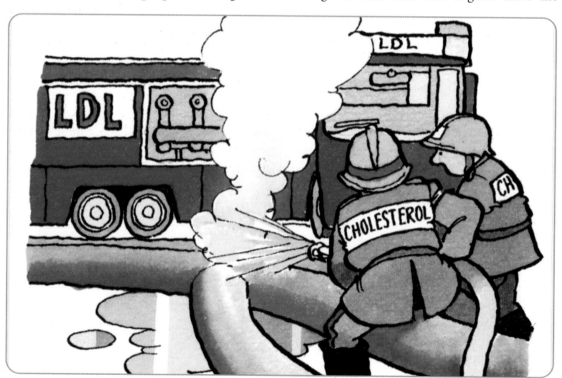

If we think of inflammation as the body on fire, cholesterol is the fire fighter and LDL is the fire engine

scene. However, if you put out the fire, then in most cases the firefighters and their engines will leave on their own.

Addressing the causes of inflammation in the body is a good strategy for reducing cardiovascular-disease risk. For elevated homocysteine levels, addressing B-vitamin deficiencies is crucial.

C-Reactive protein

There are other new markers for inflammation and cardiovascular disease including testing for C-Reactive protein (CRP) levels, which indicates a clumping of platelets or thick blood which also causes cardiovascular disease, and testing for Lipoprotein (a) which is a sticky adhesion protein. The important consideration here is that merely measuring cholesterol and lipoprotein levels is not a completely accurate predictor of cardiovascular disease. It is important to consider other factors, such as inflammation. It is also important to keep in mind that your body strives to keep its systems in balance.

Other causes of inflammation

Other causes of inflammation include blood-sugar dysregulation leading to insulin resistance and Type 2 Diabetes, allergies, stress and exposure to toxicity. See Chapter 6 for a discussion on blood sugar and Chapter 11 for a discussion on the immune system.

High blood pressure

High blood pressure (hypertension) can be caused by a number of different factors, including blockage of the arteries caused by plaque build-up, stress, smoking, hormones out of balance, being overweight and, for some people, a diet with too much salt. Hypertension is known as the silent killer because there are often no outward symptoms. The best way to find out about your blood pressure is to get it checked regularly. In the UK, the acceptable level of blood pressure is considered to be between 100/70 and 130/85 (though some people have blood pressure as low as 90/60 and are still perfectly healthy). Hypertension is a problem because it wears out blood vessels and we have blood vessels everywhere in the body.

There are some factors for having high blood pressure over which you have no control, including heredity and age, but there are many factors that you can control. If you have high blood pressure you can work at bringing it down by addressing these factors: smoking, exercise, diet, avoiding toxicity and losing weight if you need to.

Nutritional help for heart health

Here are some dietary and lifestyle suggestions for heart health.

First, use your DAL record (see Chapter 6) to record several days of your eating and activity habits. Here are some questions to help you:

- Do the foods you eat regularly contain preservatives, colourings and high levels of salt?

- Do you get regular exercise? If so, how much and how often?

- Do you smoke?

- Do you drink alcohol? If so, how much and how often?

- Does your diet contain sugar and refined carbohydrates?

You can also incorporate the following suggestions:

❧ Follow the general guidelines for a healthier diet as outlined in Chapter 1.

❧ Include healthy fats in your diet and avoid unhealthy fats. Be certain to include foods that have the Omega-3 fats. Avoid hydrogenated fats and trans fats. Refer to Chapter 2.

❧ Not everyone's blood pressure is adversely affected by sodium. If you have high blood pressure, you could try reducing your sodium intake for a while to see if your blood pressure goes down. Choose a good-quality sea salt rather than regular supermarket salt.

❧ Drink Vital Vegetable Broth (see Chapter 1) regularly. It is high in natural vegetable potassium, which helps to balance sodium in the body.

❧ Avoid oxidised or damaged cholesterol in processed foods, such as powdered eggs and milk.

❧ If you drink alcohol, it is better to limit yourself to one drink (one small glass of wine or a single measure of spirits) per day.

❧ Emphasise foods that are high in antioxidants; vitamins A, C and E and the mineral selenium. Also include foods with the B-vitamins, especially vitamin B12, vitamin B6 and folic acid. These nutrients help to reduce inflammation in the body.

❧ Fresh celery and garlic are helpful in cardiovascular disease, especially for hypertension.

❧ Make exercise a part of your daily routine, but don't overdo it.

❧ If you smoke, please stop!

This is one of the only places in this book you will see a supplement recommended, but this one is very important for heart health, especially if you have been given statin drugs to lower your cholesterol levels. Statins deplete your body of coenzyme Q10. It is a very useful supplement to support cardiovascular health. Consult a nutritional therapist to determine how to use it.

FAQs

I am on several different medications for cardiovascular disease. Are there nutrients I should not take because of a possible interaction with the drugs?
Yes, there are. If you are taking vitamin E and fish oil supplements you should check with your doctor because these have blood-thinning qualities (which can be good, but not if your medications do this as well. Eating foods such as fish or nuts should not be a problem). Anyone on prescription medication should also ask their doctor about grapefruit as there are some interactions between a substance found in grapefruit and some medications. To be safe, when your doctor prescribes any medication it's best to tell them about any supplements you are taking in case there is reason you should stop.

I have heard that some spices are good for the heart. Is this true?
Yes. There are a number of spices that are good for digestion and which also have anti-inflammatory qualities. These include turmeric, ginger, cumin and coriander. By all means, make a curry.

the immune system

This chapter looks at the immune system and how it protects you from pathogens in the environment outside your body and from damaged cells inside your body. Some foods may challenge the health of your immune system. You will be given guidelines on how to keep your immune system healthy, but you will also learn about specific problems with the immune system that are directly related to diet.

How your immune system protects you

Your immune system is always on alert. It surveys your internal environment on a 'search and destroy' mission, ensuring that if any potentially harmful organisms invade, they are quickly eliminated. It protects you from pathogens such as harmful bacteria, yeasts, fungi or parasites which may be present in the food you eat, and from harmful viruses that you may breathe in. It also protects you from any of your own cells that are not working properly, such as those that may change and become cancer cells. Your immune system sends out cells that act as scouts, analysing anything they meet as either 'self' (those cells that are a good part of you) or 'non-self' (anything that may harm you) and when they identify anything they believe is 'non-self', they summon other cells to destroy it.

Antibodies and antigens

Within your immune system there are also other cells which are more experienced, educated cells. These cells have previously met some diseases. They retain information about them and instruct their 'assistant' cells to develop antibodies to these diseases. Antibodies search for specific antigens, which are markers on cells that identify them. In a way, antigens are like little name tags that identify the cells.

For example, you might imagine that a pathogen has entered your body, and the antigen's name tag says: 'Hello, my name is nasty bug.' This may seem an odd thing for the non-self pathogen to do when it is trying to invade your body, but that is more or less what happens. Antibodies can each only help to destroy one kind of 'non-self' antigen. They do this by binding with the antigen they know, and then they control it, or they call on other immune cells to kill it. So, for this more specific part of your immune system to work against the invading nasty bug, you would need to have an antibody that recognises the name tag 'nasty bug'. This is one of the reasons breastfeeding is good for a baby: a mother can pass antibodies she has to her child in this way.

The location of your immune system

Your immune system is everywhere in your body, but there are some areas that are more concentrated parts of the immune system than others. These areas are those parts of your body where it is most likely that pathogens will enter. Your skin, which covers your entire body, is a first line of defence. It is sometimes

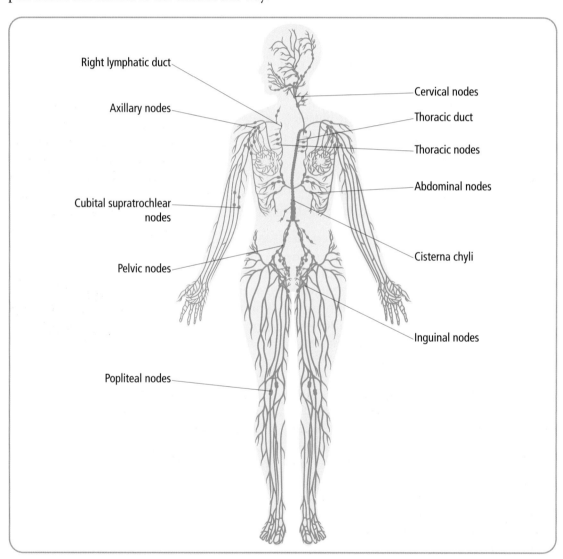

The lymph system in the body

called your 'acid mantle'. This is because healthy skin has a low level of acidity to it and this acidity is a barrier against certain pathogens. Stomach acid is an effective barrier against many pathogens due to its high level of acidity. Your small intestine has special areas that detect foreign antigens and stop pathogens from entering through its walls and getting into the inner environment of your body.

The lymph system

The lymph system is a second circulatory system in the body. It clears wastes from the system, especially the waste that results from a fight between immune cells and a non-self invader. Your lymph system literally 'removes your rubbish'.

Your liver, spleen, bone marrow and thymus gland also have immune activity. These are all examples of parts of your immune system.

Nutrition and the immune system

It is very important to keep your immune system healthy so that it can protect you from harm. Good nutrition plays a crucial role in enhancing the health of your immune system. In terms of diet, keeping your immune system healthy is just as much about what foods act as suppressors to your immune system as it is about what foods enhance its health.

Sugar and the immune system

One of the most problematic foods for the immune system is sugar. Sugar actively suppresses the immune system. In *Total Wellness*, Joseph Pizzorno (1998) describes how eating only 100 grams of sugar at one sitting suppresses the immune system within 30 minutes and how this suppression lasts for up to five hours! When you stop and think about how much sugar we typically eat every day, you may begin to realise how much of an impact you could have on the health of your immune system if you stopped eating sugar. Some people believe that honey is a better alternative, but this is only the case if the honey is raw. If it has been pasteurised, then it is similar in effect

to ordinary table sugar. Raw honey and Grade B maple syrup are better choices than table sugar, but they should be consumed in very small amounts. (If you can find it, Grade B maple syrup is less refined than Grade A and is darker in colour.) Fruit juices are not much better. Fruit juices provide a concentrated source of sugar, and you do not get the benefit

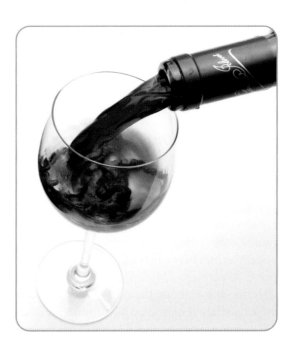

111

of the fibre from the fruit, as it has been discarded. If you must drink fruit juice, limit your amount, add some water to it if you can and make sure that it is 100 per cent fruit juice (not just a small percentage of juice from fruit with additional sugar or syrup added to it).

Simple carbohydrates and the immune system

Alcohol in excess and refined foods are other forms of simple carbohydrates similar to sugar that are not beneficial for your immune system. Alcohol does not add nutritional value to your diet and can deplete your body of stored nutrients. An exception, in small amounts, is red wine. Some studies have shown the benefits of drinking red wine because it contains a substance called resveratrol. Resveratrol acts as an antioxidant and has been shown to be protective against heart disease and some cancers. The caveat here, though, is that this protection seems only to be offered if you are drinking no more than one glass of red wine per day. Any alcohol in excess has a detrimental effect on health.

Those people who cannot drink alcohol,

such as those with have a history of alcohol abuse or those with liver disease, would not benefit from drinking red wine.

Bad fats and heart disease

The other major category of foods that suppress the immune system is bad fats. In Chapter 2 you learned that there are healthy fats and unhealthy fats. The unhealthy fats, such as the hydrogenated and trans fats, can also adversely affect your immune system.

Wholefoods and the immune system

Your immune system will respond well to a wholefood diet generally because these foods provide an array of nutrients. This will be especially true if you eat organic foods. Foods that are extra-supportive to your immune system are those which are high in antioxidants, such as vegetables and fruit: think about eating a rainbow of colours of these foods.

Food allergies and sensitivities

So far, these nutritional recommendations have been general and can apply to everyone. However, there are also some special circumstances where special nutrition recommendations can be made that will support the immune system. The first of these conditions is food allergies and food sensitivities. A food allergy exists when an individual consumes a food and their immune system erroneously identifies the food as an invading pathogen. Most people who have food allergies know about them. Allergies provoke an immediate response by the immune system. This response can be merely annoying, such as

would be the case with itching or the development of hives, or it can be life-threatening. You may know someone who has a severe allergy to peanuts. This is a common food allergy and it can be life-threatening to some people. If susceptible people eat a peanut, their throats may swell to the point where they cannot breathe. They must get to a hospital immediately for treatment.

Much less severe, but still a problem, are food sensitivities. Food sensitivities are like an allergic response, but they are not necessarily immediate. It can also be difficult to identify them because in addition to being a delayed response by the immune system, a food sensitivity response might be a symptom that most people would not associate with a food, such as migraines, fatigue, joint pain, PMT or even depression. (This is not to say that all these problems are due to food sensitivities, but they can be.) To make it even more difficult to identify food sensitivities, the reaction to a food can occur as much as several days after the food has been eaten.

If a food causes an allergic response in someone, that food is toxic to that person. In Chapter 5 you learned about toxins. Toxins are substances that are toxic to everyone. If you have a food allergy or sensitivity, that particular food is a toxin to you.

The Dietary and Lifestyle record (DAL)

How can you identify a food that might be toxic for you? There are laboratory tests that can determine allergies. You can build a very useful picture of your reaction to foods by keeping a daily dietary and lifestyle record (DAL). (You will find a blank copy of this record in Chapter 6.) If you are diligent enough to keep this record in detail every day for several weeks, you will collect some very useful information. If you are unsure how to interpret the information, consult a nutritional therapist. A nutritional therapist would look for patterns of reactions associated with the consumption of specific foods.

casestudy: Gail and green beans

Gail, 26, complained of frequent severe migraines. She had been prescribed medication, but it was not very helpful. After taking her case history, I decided to ask her to keep a DAL record for two weeks. I asked her to be very specific about listing the foods and drinks she consumed, along with the exact times she ate and drank and how she felt during the day. I asked her to use one page of the DAL record per day. When Gail returned a couple of weeks later, I looked at her records to see when her migraines occurred. Then I checked to see if there were any foods she was consuming within several days before her migraines. I had enough information to notice that every time she got a migraine she had eaten green beans two days before getting her migraine. There are many different reasons for getting migraines. In Gail's case, her immune system considered green beans to be a pathogen and it mounted a defence against the green beans, which resulted in her migraines. When Gail stopped eating green beans, she stopped getting migraines. The key to the discovery was Gail. She was very diligent about completing her dietary intake records and was very exact in her information. Green beans do not commonly cause food allergies or sensitivities, so the DAL record was our best bet in identifying that this food was a problem for Gail.

Problem foods

A toxin is something that is a poison for everyone. A food antigen is not a toxin for everyone, but for the person who has the allergy or sensitivity to it, it is a toxin. There are some foods that cause problems more often than others. These foods are:

- gluten (the protein in certain grains such as wheat)

- dairy

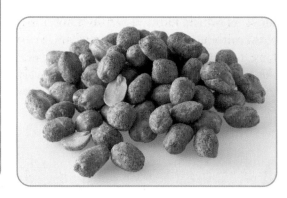

ꙍ soya

ꙍ corn

ꙍ peanuts

ꙍ eggs

ꙍ shellfish

ꙍ chocolate.

Gluten: a problem for many people

The most common food sensitivity is to gluten. Gluten is the protein found in wheat and, to a lesser degree, in other grains. These other grains include barley, rye and spelt. Sometimes oats are a problem because they are often processed in the same facility as wheat and can have wheat residue on them. It is probably easier to identify grains that do not contain gluten: these are rice, amaranth, millet and quinoa. Gluten intolerance ranges from mild sensitivity to a full-blown allergic response. The latter is called coeliac disease. If you had coeliac disease, also known as 'coeliac sprue', you would know about it because eating a food with gluten would make you very ill immediately. If a person with gluten intolerance eats foods with gluten, they have ongoing inflammation in their small intestine all the time. When this happens, the villi of the small intestine atrophy and die off. (See Chapter 5 for a discussion about villi). The villi are where our nutrients are absorbed into our inner environment, so someone with a gluten intolerance is not absorbing their nutrients well. Symptoms of a gluten intolerance can include the obvious gastro-intestinal symptoms such as diarrhoea, gas, pain, bloating or fullness but they can also include other symptoms such as joint pain, fatigue, an inability to concentrate, bone pain and ME.

Often a dairy intolerance is associated with a gluten intolerance because the enzyme to digest milk sugar is made in the tips of the intestinal villi. All this is not good news to those of you who like your toast with butter in the morning, I know!

Who is often the most gluten-intolerant

Gluten intolerance is also genetically linked and is most often found in those of British, Irish and Northern European descent. Gluten is difficult to avoid because wheat flour is a hidden ingredient in many food products as it is commonly used as a thickener. For example, you might not expect to find wheat gluten in mayonnaise or ketchup, but it might be there.

Doing a challenge test

If you suspect you might be gluten-intolerant and want to find out, you can try a challenge test. You can do this for any food you suspect you might have a sensitivity to, but you will need to test only one food at a time. To do a food challenge, you need to avoid the food you are challenging: you must not eat any of it for the entire week. While you do this, keep very detailed DAL records. Note how you feel throughout the day as well as what you are eating and drinking. You will want to follow a wholefood diet and avoid any processed foods during this time, because it is almost impossible to know what all the ingredients in processed foods are. The food you are challenging might be an unlisted ingredient in some processed foods. At the end of the week, eat the food you are challenging at breakfast and at lunch for that day and see if you have a reaction. After avoiding the food for a week, if you are sensitive to it, it is very likely that you will have a reaction. The most common reactions are flu-like symptoms, extreme fatigue, bloating, a feeling of fullness and headaches. Some people have been eating foods to which they are sensitive for many years, without realising it. Some of my clients have told me that once they have identified their problem food and avoided it for a while, they have more energy and vibrancy than they have ever had before in their lives.

A gluten experiment

In addition to being a common food allergy, gluten is also very difficult to digest. To illustrate this, you can try this simple experiment: take some bread flour and add enough water to be able to knead it into a ball of dough. Now take this dough and hold it under running tap water while you work it with your hands. Milky water will flow out of it. This is the carbohydrate starch leaving the dough. After a few minutes, you will be left with an extremely sticky gluey mass. This is the gluten or protein that is in wheat. Now imagine your digestive enzymes trying to get into this mass to digest it and break it down. Some vegetarians use gluten meat as a meat substitute in recipes. If you are vegetarian, wholefoods such as beans, legumes, grains and nuts and seeds are healthier choices.

Cravings and food sensitivities

One clue to identifying possible problem foods is to see if there are foods that you crave. Sadly, the foods we crave are often the foods we may have a sensitivity to. But if you have identified that you have a food sensitivity and you then stay off this food, you can notice a real change for the positive in your health and wellbeing. Food sensitivities are also one of the reasons why people trying to lose weight find they are unable to do so.

Inflammation and leaky gut

Consuming a food you have a sensitivity to can cause inflammation in your small intestine. Ongoing inflammation in the small intestines can cause a situation known as 'leaky gut'. Inflammation blocks nutrients from being absorbed. With a leaky gut, the walls of the small intestine become more permeable than they normally are. This allows particles which are normally too large to be able to pass through the intestinal walls to get into the blood stream. When this happens, the alert immune system will detect these particles and diagnose them as being 'non-self' and it will attack them as if they were pathogens. For

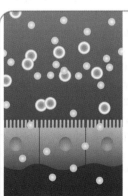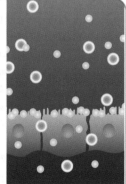

normal lining of the small intestine where nutrients pass through the lining and toxins are blocked

with leaky gut, nutrients are blocked and toxins are able to enter the blood stream

How a 'leaky gut' occurs

example, such a particle might have an antigen that has a name tag that says: 'Hello, my name is corn.' An immune antibody might then say: 'Yes, well I know corn and corn is usually smaller than you are so I think you are really a pathogen and I will make sure you get attacked!' This sets up an allergy or sensitivity to corn. Healing a leaky gut and staying off corn will calm the immune system down and quell the inflammation.

In a nutshell:

Gluten-free lasagne

Most pasta is made with wheat flour. My gluten-free clients tend to miss pasta dishes the most. You can make a lasagne dish without the gluten by substituting vegetables for the pasta. Slice some aubergines, courgettes and Portobello mushrooms lengthwise to make long strips. Lay them flat on a baking sheet and lightly brush with olive oil using a pastry brush. Sprinkle a little sea salt over the vegetable slices and then bake them in a hot oven until they have dried out somewhat and are slightly browned. Now layer them with your lasagne sauce where you would normally layer the pasta sheets.

Healthy intestinal flora

Another main nutritional issue regarding the immune system is the maintenance of healthy flora (probiotics) in the intestines. Healthy flora consist of beneficial bacteria. These bacteria work for us in that they crowd out any bad bacteria that might invade our intestines, and they also crowd out yeasts and fungi. Your internal ecosystem is alive with thousands of these various microorganisms. In addition to keeping other organisms in check, the beneficial bacteria keep the body generally alkaline, which is the most beneficial pH state for good health; they maintain the health of the immune system; they aid your digestion; and they actually *make* some vitamins for you. In contrast, if you have bad bacteria in your gut, they create toxins, which can weaken your immune system and your overall health. If you have an imbalance of bad bacteria, yeasts and fungi over the good bacteria, this is called dysbiosis. Some health experts believe that maintaining proper gut ecology is the best way to ensure good health.

Candida

All of us have a yeast, called candida, in our gut ecology. Normally, this yeast is neither good nor bad. But if the good bacteria are killed off, they are not available to crowd out candida yeast and keep it in check. If the playing field of your gut is somewhat empty and wide open, this yeast is free to grow in wild abandon. When it does this, it changes its form from being a yeast to a fungus, and this is when it becomes a problem. In its fungal form, candida grows long tendrils which can penetrate through the gut walls, making holes in it. This is another reason for 'leaky gut'. This of course sets up your system for the development of allergies and food sensitivities, as any large food particles passing through the leaks in the gut lining and into your bloodstream will be attacked by your immune system for being 'non-self' organisms. Candida overgrowth can be caused by a history of antibiotic usage in the past. Antibiotics are lifesaving drugs, but they have a downside. They do not discriminate between killing bad bacteria and good bacteria. Restoring healthy bacteria can take some time and diligence in sticking with a diet that strictly controls yeast. This is best done with the support of a nutritional therapist.

The rotation diet

Sometimes you can develop a food sensitivity to foods that you eat every day. Because of this, some nutritionists recommend following a rotation diet. With a rotation diet, you never eat the same food several days in a row. For example, if you have rice on Monday, you would not then have rice again until after Wednesday of the same week. This way, you might not develop a food sensitivity to rice. Following a rotation diet is especially useful if you are healing a leaky gut and are undertaking strategies to calm your immune system. Some nutritionists believe that we all should follow a rotational way of eating as a general healthy practice.

Suggestions for a healthy immune system

First, use your DAL record to record several days of your eating and activity habits. Look for answers to the following questions:

- Given the information above, do you suspect you might have a food sensitivity?
- Are there sugar or refined foods in your diet?
- Is there a food that you eat every day?

If you have answered 'Yes' to any of these questions, you might try a food-challenge test. If you think you might have a food sensitivity, or if you think you might have dysbiosis, you might consult a dietary therapist to help you design a healing therapeutic diet to address these issues. Try rotating the foods that you eat every day.

Here are some dietary and lifestyle suggestions for immune system support:

- If you have done a food-challenge test and have identified a food you suspect might be a problem for you, avoid this food for several months to allow your intestines to heal and your immune system to calm down. You can try the food again later to see if you need to stay off it for even

longer. Some people find that they feel so much better avoiding problem foods that they have no desire to eat them again. Avoiding foods that you have an intolerance to is a really key element in strengthening your immune system.

- Follow the general guidelines for a wholefood diet as outlined in Chapter 1. But avoid those foods you are intolerant of.
- Avoid sugar and sugary foods, which suppress the immune system and also feed yeast.
- If you like garlic, raw garlic is very supportive to the immune system. Garlic is antifungal, antiviral and antibacterial. When asked what one food or herb they would wish to have if stranded on a deserted island, many herbalists have said 'garlic'. A clove a day is good. If fighting an infection, a few cloves a day are better.
- If it is available to you, coconut oil is also antifungal and antiviral. Use 2–3 tablespoons of coconut oil per day, in cooking or drizzled over steamed vegetables.

- If you suspect you might have a yeast-overgrowth problem, follow the other recommendations here, and also try avoiding fermented foods and drinks such as vinegar and alcohol; also avoid fungal and bacterial foods such as mushrooms and blue cheeses.

- The short-chain fatty acids are supportive of the immune system. These would be included in foods such as butter, which has butyric acid in it. (See Chapter 2 on fats.) Ghee (clarified butter used in Indian cooking) is also a good choice. Remember to eat these sparingly. For immune support, strictly avoid hydrogenated fats.

- Vitamin C and zinc are well-known for being supportive to the immune system. Refer to Chapter 3 for food sources of these nutrients.

- Sea vegetables (available in healthfood stores) are very high in minerals that will help to strengthen the immune system. A great way to start using them is to place a strip of kombu in every pot of beans, stew or soup that you cook. You can remove it before serving the meal and the minerals will remain in the food.

- If you are eating grains or beans, it is really important to follow the instructions on enhancing digestion of these foods found in Chapter 1.

FAQs

I know that probiotics can be given in supplemental form. Are these good to take?

Generally the best way to enhance your healthy flora is to discourage the pathogenic bacteria and yeast and feed the beneficial bacteria. Sugar and heavy protein eating feed the pathogenic organisms. You can feed and nourish your healthy bacteria by following the dietary guidelines in Chapter 5. Probiotic supplements can be used therapeutically for a short period of time but it is better to 'grow' your own healthy bacteria. Also, make sure you have enough fibre in your diet.

I drink probiotic drinks and eat a lot of yogurt. Will this help to provide my body with healthy bacteria?

Read the labels on the drinks carefully. They may have some healthy bacteria but they can also contain a lot of sugar. This negates the purpose of consuming the probiotics because sugar feeds yeast. The same is true for many yogurts.

If I think I have a food sensitivity and I try to stay off this food for a while to let my immune system calm down, will I ever be able to eat this food again?

It depends. In some cases, people find that after staying off the food for a while they can reintroduce it later on with no problem, as long as they don't eat it every day. However, other people find that when they re-introduce the food they still have a problem with it and need to stay off it. Keeping detailed DAL records during this time will help you to determine if you can eat the food again or if you still need to avoid it. If you have a true allergy, however, you must stay off the food. If you are unsure about identifying any food intolerances, consult a nutritional therapist.

ageing and the skin

In this chapter you will learn about how nutrition can be beneficial for your skin and can therefore help you to look healthy.

You will learn that beauty is not only about what you put on your skin, but is enhanced by the foods you eat.

Anti-ageing

'Anti-ageing' is a buzzword in health circles. So many of us want to look younger, be more vibrant and have more energy. 'Growing old gracefully' has given way to 'turning back the clock'. But the reality is that you can't turn back the clock. Time moves forward and so do we. Your best bet for looking younger in the long run is to aim to incorporate healthy nutrition and lifestyle practices and to back them up with natural skin care. Chapter 5 covers the subject of toxicity. Skin products loaded with chemicals are another source of toxicity. (You can learn more about this in another book in this series: *Aromatherapy in Essence*.)

Skin

Your skin is the largest organ of your body. The liver is the major organ of detoxification, but your skin also plays a major role in the detoxification process. Some toxicity can be released through the skin in the form of sweat or skin eruptions. So, enhancing your overall internal health by reducing exposure to toxicity will also enhance the health and appearance of your skin.

As you saw in Chapter 11, your skin's acid mantle performs an important function as part of your immune system. The health of your skin reflects your overall health. In fact, in Oriental medicine, skin diagnosis is a very important way of diagnosing what is going on in the body. Your food choices are reflected in the health of your skin. These practitioners can tell from examining your skin whether or not you ate sugar earlier that day! Your skin tells a story about your current state of health. It goes through changes: it can be dry, moist, pale, dark or inflamed. It might develop a rash, turn yellowish in colour, break out in spots, itch, burn, or become prematurely wrinkled. All of these events are signs of what is going on inside you.

Free radicals

Your skin cells are always dying off and are being replaced by new cells. This means that you have an opportunity to enhance the character of your skin by enhancing your general health, so that as you replace old cells with new cells the new cells will be healthy cells. One of skin's greatest enemies is the inflammation caused by free radical damage. Free radicals age your body faster than anything.

Free radicals are molecules that are incomplete because they are missing an electron. They roam your body, seeking to be complete. Electrons are tiny particles that are negatively charged. Free radicals are usually created through the process of burning oxygen. Your own metabolism naturally does this, so you make your own free radicals just by living, breathing and metabolising. A free radical's mission is to find an electron it can steal and make its own. Unfortunately, it will steal electrons from places such as your own DNA, red blood cells or cell membranes.

Because free radicals are produced as a by-product of normal metabolism, your body has the ability to deal with them.

Inflammation and oxidative stress

Unfortunately, you are not only exposed to the free radicals that your body makes as a by-product of your own metabolism. Inflammation in your body also causes the production of free radicals. Exposure to toxicity such as environmental pollution and radiation also creates free radicals. Radiation exposure includes that which you get from too much sun exposure. Because oxygen is initially involved in the process of free radical creation, the damage that free radicals do is called oxidative stress, though there are other causes as well. Don't think of oxygen as the 'baddie', though. It is necessary for life! A better description might be to think of oxidative stress as a form of rusting inside. Think about seeing something that has been left outside in the rain and weather. It looks old, doesn't it?

If you look at it this way, you can understand why exposure to oxidative stress is ageing. One of the worst sources of chemicals that generate free radicals is cigarette smoke. You can often see the damage that it has done in the faces of people who smoke a lot. Their skin is often prematurely aged and wrinkled. This is because free radicals have damaged the collagen in their skin.

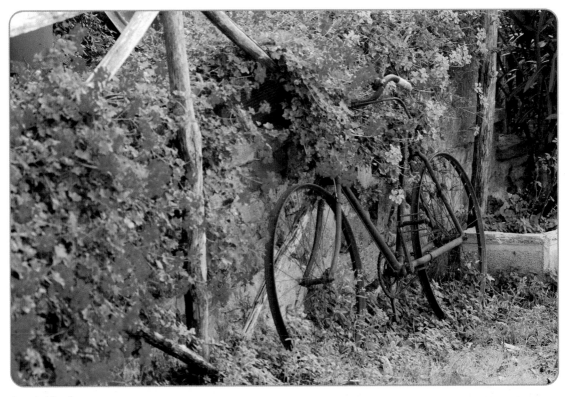

A rusty bicycle

In a nutshell:

Grated cauliflower with Indian spices

Spices such as ginger and turmeric have anti-inflammatory properties. Try this Indian spiced dish as a part of your strategy for youthful skin.
200 grms of the grated head of a cauliflower (see below)

150g of fresh or frozen peas, steamed and strained
20g of ginger, grated
1 clove of garlic, grated
½ tsp cumin seeds
½ tsp turmeric powder

2 tsp of cardamom powder
½ tsp of sea salt
½ tsp teaspoon of garam masala
80 cl of coconut oil

1 Use a cheese grater to grate the head of a cauliflower. Reserve 200 grms of this for this recipe.
2 Heat the coconut oil and add the cumin seeds. Be careful not to burn the seeds, and sauté them until they begin to pop.
3 Add the ginger, garlic, cauliflower, peas, turmeric, salt and garam masala.
4 Mix well, cover and sauté for 7 minutes.
5 Mix in the cardamom powder and serve.

Antioxidants

How can you counteract the damage done by oxidative stress? Apart from reducing your exposure to pollutants such as cigarette smoke, you can include foods in your diet that contain the antioxidant nutrients. The best-known antioxidant nutrients are vitamin A and beta-carotene, vitamin C, vitamin E and the mineral selenium. The antioxidants work in conjunction with each other so it is best to include all of them together. Antioxidants travel around your body and donate one of their electrons to each free radical that is seeking one. When they do this, the free radicals stop their tissue damage. Antioxidants regenerate each other and this is why it is best to include all of them in your diet.

Phytochemicals and flavonoids in plant foods

Various plant chemicals also contain antioxidants, even though they are not vitamins or minerals. These chemicals are called phytochemicals. Phytochemicals give you powerful protection against oxidative stress. Their protection is so powerful, it is thought that phytochemicals are the reason a plant-based diet is so good for your health. These phytochemicals are protective against cancer and other degenerative diseases. There

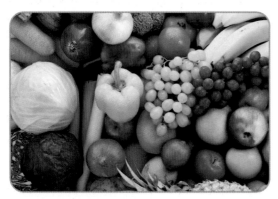

Fruit and vegetables contain phytochemicals

are many different phytochemicals and they are related to the pigments in fruits and vegetables.

This is why it is a good idea to think of a rainbow when choosing these foods. The orange in carrots, apricots and pumpkin; the red of tomatoes and cherries; the green of avocadoes and leafy greens; the brown in nuts and seeds; and the blue found in blueberries are examples of these pigments. All of these foods contain phytochemicals. Coincidentally, these foods also contain vitamins A (as beta-carotene), C, E and selenium as well. You may be familiar with the term 'flavonoids'. Flavonoids are examples of phytochemicals. A diet rich with foods containing antioxidants will help you to have healthy, glowing skin.

Essential fats

A good balance of the essential fats is also important for skin health.

Please note that essential fats are not the same as essential oils. Essential fats are dietary fats. For more about essential fats, refer to Chapter 2. Essential oils are used in aromatherapy. For more about essential oils, refer to *Aromatherapy In Essence*.

Eating a diet that is extremely low in fat or that contains no fat will result in skin that is more dry and wrinkled. That is because it is deficient in the essential fats. You need an array of healthy fats in your diet to keep your skin moist and supple. In addition to including healthy fats, it is important to exclude unhealthy fats. These include hydrogenated fats and trans fats. Polyunsaturated fats, such as the vegetable oils, are very subject to becoming damaged and rancid. These fats are especially damaged if they are used in frying. When this happens and you consume these fats, you are getting a lot of free radicals in your diet. It is best to avoid any fats that have been damaged.

Grocery-store vegetable oils are especially vulnerable to this damage as they are highly processed using heat, and they are usually stored in clear plastic bottles under bright lights. Polyunsaturated fats are easily damaged by heat, light and oxygen. See Chapter 2 for more on healthy and unhealthy fats.

Dehydration

Dehydration is another reason for dry skin. Your body contains between 60 and 70 per cent water. Since you lose water through urine, sweat and your breath, it is important to replenish lost water. Though some researchers have recently claimed that increasing water intake has no effect on the appearance of skin, many people have found this not to be the case. Water not only rehydrates your body, it helps to flush out toxicity. For more information on the benefits of water, see Chapter 4.

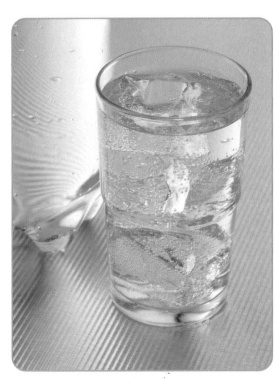

Water hydrates the body and helps flush out toxins

Ageing and sugar

Sugar and refined processed foods contribute to advanced ageing because they can lead to unbalanced blood-sugar levels. Processed foods often contain chemicals such as artificial colourings and preservatives. Your body needs to detoxify these chemicals

Refined foods can lead to insulin resistance. Insulin resistance is an inflammatory condition and results in the creation of many free radicals. See Chapter 6 for a discussion on insulin resistance.

Sugar and refined carbohydrates can cause another problem. Glucose that is not used for energy or stored as fat can attach itself to proteins in your body. This process is called glycation and these sugary proteins are called advanced glycated end products, or more appropriately, 'AGES', which is what they do. These sugary proteins are very inflammatory.

Food allergies and sensitivities are also a cause of inflammation. Identifying these and avoiding the foods you have a problem with will help to reduce free radical formation. See Chapter 11 for a discussion on allergies and food sensitivities.

The lymph system

Assisting your lymph system to work properly is a good strategy to employ if you want to look younger and healthier. (You first read about the lymph system in Chapter 11). Your lymph system is a network of vessels, like your circulatory system, that flows through your body. Lymph is the fluid that flows through these vessels. Lymph consists of fluid that comes from spaces between your cells. It collects any waste products from metabolic activities that have taken place within your cells. It parallels your circulatory system through most of your body: fluid is exchanged between the two systems. Dotted along these lymph vessels are lymph nodes. Lymph nodes contain cells of your immune system that monitor the lymph that flows through them, seeking out and destroying any pathogens that are contained in the lymph. You will know where some of these nodes are when you are ill because they become inflamed and swollen as they are fighting pathogens. The most noticeable of the lymph nodes are at the sides of your neck, under your jaw. Think of your lymph system as a cleanser: it takes out your rubbish for you.

Unlike your circulatory system, which uses your pumping heart for assistance, your lymph system does not have an organ to help the lymph move around your body. The only way the lymph can move is when your muscles help to push it through. The primary muscle that does this is your diaphragm, which expands when you breathe and squeezes the major lymph vessels to push lymph through. This is one reason why breathing exercises are helpful for your health.

The lymph system and exercise

Exercise is another way that you can enhance your lymph flow. By getting regular exercise, you allow your contracted muscles to squeeze and push lymph through your body. One of the best exercises is rebounding. A rebounder is a mini-trampoline that allows you to jump as you would if you were skipping rope, but to do so without putting any stress on your joints. Walking is another form of beneficial exercise that is not stressful to your body. Manual lymph drainage is a form of massage

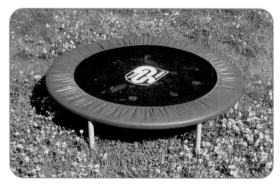

A rebounder

therapy where the therapist helps you to move your lymph by using specific massage strokes.

Dry-skin brushing

Dry-skin brushing is beneficial for the lymph system. It also helps to keep the skin fresh and glowing, as it removes dead cells and allows new ones to breathe.

Dry-skin brushing is a routine practice of brushing the dry skin off the body for about 3–5 minutes, usually done in the morning before a shower or bath. It is invigorating, stimulates both blood and lymph circulation and removes old dead cells. Daily brushing can lead to soft, glowing, fresh-looking skin and can have an invigorating effect on the body. In stimulating circulation, which nourishes our entire system, dry-skin brushing may also help to reduce the appearance of cellulite because it brings the circulation to the affected area. Some sources say that five minutes of brushing is as good in contributing to physical tone as 30 minutes of jogging. You might even find that you don't need that morning cup of coffee to wake you up if you follow this routine!

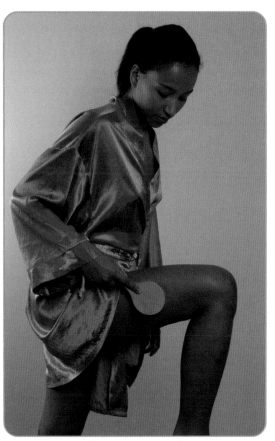

Dry skin brushing

How to dry-skin-brush

You will need a natural bristle or plant-fibre long-handled brush, which is not to be shared with anyone else (in the same way that you wouldn't share a toothbrush). The head of the brush should be about the size of your hand, and the handle should be long enough to allow you to get at hard-to-reach places, such as the middle of your back. Do not use a brush with synthetic bristles (e.g. nylon). Most healthfood stores carry dry skin brushes. The entire skin-brushing routine should take about 3–5 minutes. Every couple of weeks, clean your brush as you would a hairbrush, and allow it to dry in a ventilated place. Dry-skin brushes usually have a hole in the handle to hang them up with.

To dry-skin-brush, start at the soles of your feet and then move up to your toes, feet and ankles. Brush the front and back of your legs. Always move upwards towards your heart, making upward sweeping strokes. Your brush strokes should be strong enough to encourage circulation to the area and make it a healthy pink, but not so strong that your skin is damaged in any way. At your abdomen, make anti-clockwise circular movements, which is brushing in the direction of the colon's natural movement. Brush your back and chest upwards toward your heart. Brush your fingers, hands, elbows and arms, also in the direction of your heart. Finally, brush your neck, upper back and upper chest downwards towards your heart.

> Note – People with extremely delicate or easily damaged skin might find this process challenging. Skin brushing should never be done over an open wound or over large, raised moles. If there are known malignancies of the skin or lymph system, these are also contraindications. If you have an inflammatory rash, allow this to heal first before attempting to dry-skin-brush. The face, large varicose veins, the genital area and nipples are sensitive areas of the body that are avoided in dry-skin brushing.

After dry-skin brushing

Some people like to take an invigorating shower to wash off the exfoliated cells and also to increase tone and circulation. Hot and cold showering can be a very effective way to further stimulate the circulation. To do this, take a hot shower for 2–3 minutes and then follow this with a cold shower for 20 seconds. Repeat this process of hot followed by cold several times. This type of hydrotherapy is believed to reduce an over-acidic system and boost the endocrine system.

Skin conditions

Let's look at some specific conditions where nutrition can help to improve the health and appearance of the skin.

Cellulite

Cellulite is the bumpy skin that occurs when the supportive tissues in your skin become weak and allow fat cells to move around. Good skin health can help to control cellulite. Vitamin C is an important nutrient for skin, as are all the antioxidants. Massage therapy with essential oils is also beneficial. See *Aromatherapy in Essence* for suggestions.

Eczema

Eczema is a skin inflammation that is very much linked to food allergies. Identifying possible problem foods and eliminating them from your diet will help enormously with this problem. Gluten, dairy, peanuts and eggs are the most common problem foods, but remember that anyone can be intolerant of any food substance. See Chapter 11 for a discussion of food sensitivities.

Acne

There are several underlying causes of acne. Hormonal imbalances are a likely culprit. Since sugar and refined foods can lead to insulin resistance or high levels of insulin in the blood, eliminating these foods and focusing on a wholefood diet can be helpful. Acne can also be related to an imbalance of fats and a deficiency of the essential fats in the diet.

Suggestions for healthy skin

Here are some dietary and lifestyle suggestions for keeping your skin healthy and for looking younger through health.

First, use your DAL record (See Chapter 6) to record several days of your eating and activity habits. Look for answers to the following questions:

- Are there sugar or refined foods in your diet?
- Do you see any foods that you believe you may be sensitive to?
- Are you incorporating good healthy fats in your diet?
- Could you be dehydrated?

If you have answered 'Yes' to any of these questions, here are some suggestions to enhance the health of your skin and to help you look younger by being healthier.

Follow the general guidelines for a wholefoods diet as outlined in Chapter 1.

- To avoid ongoing inflammation, identify any possible food intolerances and avoid these foods.
- Avoid sugar and refined carbohydrates as these lead to blood-sugar imbalances and advanced glycated end products (AGES).
- Consider some of the detoxification strategies outlined in Chapter 5.
- Eliminating toxins can help create healthy skin.
- Include healthy fats in your diet and avoid fats such as hydrogenated and trans fats (see Chapter 2). Avoid heavily fried foods. Coconut oil is an oil that helps create silky skin when it is used both internally and

externally. Also incorporate a little olive oil in cooking.

- Ginger is a spice that has anti-inflammatory properties. Try incorporating fresh ginger in your diet. Try a ginger tea: Put slices of fresh ginger into a tea cup. Add boiling water and let it steep for a few minutes before removing the ginger slices. Add some lemon juice. (Turmeric also has some anti-inflammatory properties. Try the recipe in the 'In a nutshell' section of this chapter.)

- Increase your intake of non-dehydrating fluids if you are not drinking enough.

- Increase your intake of foods that contain antioxidants and phytochemicals. These are primarily vegetables, fruits, nuts and seeds. If you like it, green tea has also been shown to have antioxidant

properties. Drink it in moderation, as it does also contain some caffeine.

- Support your lymph system by incorporating one or more of the following in your daily routine: rebounding or another form of exercise, and dry-skin brushing.

- Getting adequate sleep helps to restore the body. New cells are regenerated during times of sleep. You know the saying: ' I am getting my beauty sleep.'

- If you are under a lot of stress, try to incorporate stress-management techniques. Refer to *Stress Management in Essence* for suggestions on how to do this.

- Consider getting regular massage with essential oils, or having manual lymph drainage massage.

127

FAQs

I have rosacea. What nutritional strategies can you suggest for this skin condition?
First, use your DAL (See Chapter 6) to try to identify food intolerances. If you can identify the foods that irritate you, try eliminating them for a while. Also consider eliminating sugar, caffeine, alcohol, hydrogenated fats (and other foods identified in Chapter 11), which are the most common allergens. Make sure you include the healthy fats in your diet and drink plenty of filtered water. Eat vegetables and fruit and make sure your diet is plant-based.

I have terrible cellulite on my thighs. Can you help?
Cellulite consists of fat deposits just below the surface of the skin. (Read this chapter for more on cellulite.) Apart from ensuring that your circulation is healthy through regular exercise, you can try dry-skin brushing and hot and cold showering. Nutritionally, look more toward attaining a good balance of the healthy essential dietary fats and eliminate refined foods and sugar. As mentioned, also include some foods that are high in vitamin C in your diet.

My skin has a dull, yellowish and almost grey cast to it. I have been to my doctor and she says I am not ill. How can I have healthier looking skin?
I am glad that you consulted your doctor. Now that you know that you don't have an underlying illness, consider giving your liver a rest: it may be overworked. You might try some gentle detoxification (see Chapter 5). If you smoke, please consider giving it up. (If you are exposed to second-hand smoke, do your best to avoid it.) If you drink alcohol, consider a break from it for a while. Preferably, cut the amount of alcohol that you drink right down. Increase your consumption of filtered water (see Chapter 4) and antioxidant-rich foods. Lower your intake of protein and ensure that you are following a plant-based diet rich with a variety of vegetables.

where to go from here

If you have enjoyed this book, learned something and had fun in the process, then it has been a success. That may be as far as you want to take it. But you may want to learn more. You have a wide variety of options at this point. You may want to:

ॐ stop here and just follow the suggestions given in the book

ॐ learn more about healthy cooking

ॐ consider formal training as a nutritional therapist

ॐ contact the author's website for information and articles of interest.

Using the suggestions in the book

The information given in *Nutrition in Essence* provides a basic understanding about the definition of wholefoods are and why they are important for health. Using the DAL form that is provided (see Chapter 6), you can record the foods you eat and how you feel throughout the day. Though this exercise may seem simple, it is a valuable source of information concerning how the foods and drinks you consume affect your health and wellbeing. For example, if you notice that you become tired after eating a particular food, you can avoid that food for a while to see if you may have an intolerance to it. The information you get from keeping a DAL will give you the power to make decisions about the food you eat.

Following the recipes

The recipes given in the book are examples of how a meal using wholefoods is not only healthy but also delicious. You can create your own recipes, using them as templates from which to create your own healthy and delicious recipes.

Finding a course in healthy wholefoods cooking

There are many courses available that teach healthy cooking: some are one-off courses centred around a specific topic, others offer a series of classes. There are many reputable courses available across the UK (too many to list here, but easy to find using the Internet).

129

From reading *Nutrition in Essence*, you will realise that there are differing opinions as to what constitutes healthy cooking.

Nutritional therapist training

Nutritional therapists evaluate and advise people regarding their diets and food plans. They are more qualified to recommend supplement therapy for individuals if needed. The minimum length of training is 2–3 years.

There are several courses available. To learn more about this type of training, you might begin by visiting the website of BANT, the professional organisation to which many nutritional therapists belong. BANT stands for The British Association for Nutritional Therapy. The website address is: www.BANT. org.uk.

At the time of writing, nutrition in clinical practice is unregulated in the UK, but most therapists who have graduated from the UK schools below join BANT.

Nutritional Therapy Schools in the UK

Plaskett Nutritional Medicine College (PNMC)

The author of *Nutrition in Essence* attended this college. PNM College is now a part of Thames Valley University. To find out more about this training, contact either website: www.pnmcollege.com or www.health.tvu. ac.uk/plaskett.

The Institute for Optimum Nutrition (ION)

ION was founded in 1984 by Patrick Holford. To find out more about this school, visit their website at: www.ion.ac.uk.

Distance learning

Hawthorn Health and Nutrition Institute

This school offers only distance-learning programmes and therefore would be appropriate for students who wish to remain in the UK but who want to study nutritional therapy at an American school. Students are connected with each other and the tutors through Hawthorn's very interactive website. The author of *Nutrition in Essence* has also attended this school. Hawthorn offers three programmes: a certified program as a Nutrition Consultant, a Master's Degree of Science in Holistic Nutrition and a Master's Degree in Health and Nutrition Education. For more information, visit the Hawthorn website at: www.hawthorninstitute.org.

The author's website

If you are interested in learning more about the various nutritional issues presented in *Nutrition in Essence*, you may like to visit the author's website at: www.rootstohealth.com.

Further reading

The following books give additional information regarding wholefoods diets and the health of indigenous peoples all over the world. Some of these books include recipes and some books also investigate the science behind the myths and truths of nutrition, as discussed in *Nutrition in Essence.*

Fallon, Sally (2001) *Nourishing Traditions* (2nd edition), New Trends Publishing Inc.

Enig, Mary G. (2000) *Know Your Fats: The Complete Primer for Understanding the Nutrition of Fats, Oils and Cholesterol,* Bethesda Press

Ravenskov, Uffe (2000) *The Cholesterol Myths* New Trends Publishing, Inc.

Price, Weston A. (2000) *Nutrition and Physical Degeneration* (14th printing), The Price-Pottinger Nutrition Foundation

Schmid, Ronald F. (1997) *Traditional Foods are Your Best Medicine,* Healing Arts Press

Prentice, Jessica (2006) *Full Moon Feast Food and the Connection to Hunger,* Chelsea Green Publishing

Katz, Rebecca (2004) *One Bite at a Time,* Celestial Arts

Schmid, Ron (2003) *The Untold Story of Milk,* New Trends Publishing, Inc.

Danieal, Kaayle T. (2005) *The Whole Soy Story,* New Trends Publishing, Inc.

Ross, Julia (1999) *The Diet Cure,* Viking Press

Batmanghelidj, F. (2003) *You're Not Sick, You're Thirsty,* Warner Books

glossary

acid mantle: A term that describes the outer, protective layer of the skin, which has a pH that is slightly acidic. It is the immune system's first line of defence against pathogens that might otherwise invade through the skin.

Advanced Glycated End Products (AGEs); glycation: When blood sugar levels are high, the circulating sugar in the blood can bind to proteins without the influence of enzymes. This process is glycation. These sugar-coated proteins (AGEs) cause inflammation and the creation of free radicals in the body. They are toxic and cause premature aging.

antibodies: Proteins produced by immune cells in the body when there are specific antigens present. Antibodies combine with antigens to neutralise or destroy them.

antigens: Any substance which, when it enters the body, causes the immune system to produce antibodies against it because the body registers the antigen as a pathogen that needs to be neutralised or destroyed.

antioxidants: Nutrients that help to protect the body against the damage caused by free radicals. These nutrients include vitamins A, C and E and the mineral selenium.

biochemical individuality: A term invented by the biochemist Roger Williams. In nutritional terms, it implies that because we all have unique nutritional needs, there is no one 'right' diet that will work for everyone.

bioflavonoids: Vitamin-like substances in foods that act as antioxidants in the body.

cardiovascular disease (CVD): Refers to a group of diseases or adverse conditions that affect the heart and the blood vessels.

carcinogenic: Describes a substance or agent, exposure to which increases the chance of developing cancer.

coeliac disease: A disease of the small intestine that is caused by an immune reaction to the gluten component found in grains such as wheat, oats, rye, spelt and kamut. Other terms for this condition include 'gluten-sensitive enteropathy' and 'nontropical sprue'.

challenge test: A home-based test where the immune response to foods is tested by withdrawing a food or substance form the diet for a week and then reintroducing that food at breakfast and lunch at the end of the week. If a reaction occurs, there may be a sensitivity or allergy to the food. It is important to challenge only one food at a time, to determine which foods cause reactions.

chelate: A molecule which can be bound to a mineral so that mineral is better absorbed into the body.

cholesterol: A substance that is found in animal foods. The liver can make cholesterol if necessary. We need some cholesterol to make hormones, including cortisol and some of the body's oestrogen and testosterone. Cholesterol only becomes dangerous if it oxidises or becomes damaged and then makes deposits in the arteries.

chyme: The term given to food once it is in the stomach and the small intestine. By this stage, the food is mostly digested and is well mixed with digestive secretions.

133

coenzymes: Substances that activate enzymes so they can work properly.

co-factors: Agents that product an effect in the body when they are joined with other agents.

C-Reactive Protein (CRP): If this substance is present in high amounts on a blood test, it indicates that there is inflammation somewhere in the body.

cultured vegetables: Vegetables to which a substance has been added to pre-digest them so that they are more easily digested by the human digestive system.

cysts: A little sac or pouch which is surrounded by a wall and which contains fluid or solid material.

dehydration: A condition that occurs when fluid intake does not keep up with loss of fluids. The most common cause is diarrhoea, but it can also occur because of low fluid intake, consuming liquids containing caffeine or alcohol (which are dehydrating), or through excessive sweat.

diabetes Types 1 and 2: A disease where there is too much sugar (glucose) in the blood because it cannot get into the cells where it would be burned for energy. The hormone insulin is needed to get glucose into the cells. Type 1 Diabetes is insulin dependent which means insulin must be taken because the body cannot make it. Type 2 Diabetes is non-insulin dependent, but glucose cannot get into the cells because they are not as responsive to insulin. Type 2 Diabetes is more linked to diet.

digestive enzymes: Enzymes in the digestive tract that help digest carbohydrates, fats and proteins in food.

diuretics: Drugs or other substances which increase the output of urine. They can deplete the body of minerals such as potassium and sodium.

double bond: In the chemical structure of fats, the area where hydrogen atoms are missing and where the fat molecule is more fluid.

dysbiosis: A state where the kind of flora in the intestines is more pathogenic or where there is too much yeast and not enough beneficial flora. The health of the body depends on having beneficial flora in the intestines.

emulsification: In nutrition, the term for when fats are broken down into smaller droplets so that the fat digestive enzymes can break them down for digestion.

endometrium: The mucous membrane that lines the uterus. It is vascular (contains blood vessels) and during menstruation, the functional layer of the endometrium is shed.

enzymes: Proteins that change the rate of chemical reactions without needing an outside energy source to do so and without being changed themselves. They only act on specific substances and work best at optimum temperatures and pH levels.

enzyme inhibitors: Substances naturally occurring on grains, nuts and seeds which inhibit the action of digestive enzymes, making these foods more difficult to digest. These inhibitors can be removed through soaking and then draining these foods.

'fight or flight' response: The stress response which readies the body to 'fight' or 'flee from' a stressor.

flora: The population of live bacteria and yeasts that live in the intestines.

food allergies and sensitivities: Situations specific to individuals where the immune systems reacts to specific foods as if they were pathogens that need to be destroyed.

free radical: A molecule which possesses a free electron which makes it unstable. A free radical will travel around the body searching for a molecule to react with, including fats, proteins, cell membranes and even your own DNA. Antioxidant molecules are like opposites to free radicals. They sacrifice themselves to join free radicals, which protects cells from damage.

ghee: Butter fat with the protein solids from butter removed. Ghee is traditionally used in India.

glucose: The form of sugar recognised by the body as a source of energy.

gluten: The protein found in many grains to which some people are sensitive. The true name of the substance in gluten that causes immune reactions is gliadin, but most people refer to it as gluten.

Glycaemic Index and Glycaemic Load:
Glycaemic Index and Glycaemic Load are two ways of considering the potential effects that the carbohydrate components of various foods have on the body. high numbers on a Glycaemic Index indicates that the food will elevate blood sugar levels quickly. But with this index, a chocolate bar and a carrot can have a similar number. Glycaemic Load takes into consideration the quality and the amount of carbohydrates in a food. With this index, the carrot would fare better nutritionally than the chocolate.

high-fructose corn syrup: This is a very sweet form of corn syrup that is very high in fructose. It is found in soft drinks and other refined products. Many health advocates believe that consumption of this refined sugar product is a significant contributing factor to the obesity and diabetes epidemics in modern society.

homocysteine: A high level of this amino acid in the blood can signify an increased risk of developing atherosclerosis. A diet rich in folic acid, and vitamins B6 and B12 can be preventative for a build up of this substance in the blood.

hypertension: A term for high blood pressure.

intrinsic factor: A substance secreted by glands in the stomach that is necessary for the absorption of vitamin B12.

lactase: The enzyme specific to the digestion of lactose.

lactose: The main sugar found in milk.

leaky gut: A term given to the condition where the semi-permeable lining of the small intestine is breached and holes developed, which allow larger particles than acceptable to the body to pass through into the bloodstream.

lipase: An enzyme specific to fat digestion.

lipoproteins, Lipoprotein(a): Proteins bound with fat which travel though the bloodstream. Some are associated with heart disease and others are associated with the prevention of heart disease. Lipoproteins transport fats to other tissues in the body. Lipoprotein a) is associated with atherosclerosis.

lycopene: An antioxidant found in tomatoes and other red fruits, including berries.

macrobiotic diet: A therapeutic diet that originated in Japan.

metabolise: The body processes of converting food molecules into body tissues and cells and of breaking down complex molecules into more simple molecules, such as the case with digestion and detoxification.

monounsaturated fats: Fatty acids that contain only one double bond.

nutrient dense: Description of foods that have greater amounts of nutrients per calorie.

oestrogen dominant A situation that occurs when oestrogen levels are high, relative to progesterone levels. This means that a woman could be in menopause and have low oestrogen levels, but she could still be oestrogen dominant because her progesterone levels are extremely low. Oestrogen dominance makes a woman more susceptible to developing oestrogen-dependent cancers such as breast cancer.

pathogens: Micro-organisms that can create disease.

phytic acid: An example of an enzyme inhibitor.

phytochemicals, phytonutrients: Substances found in plants which are not vitamins or minerals, but nutrients important in their own right. These substances are associated with protecting the body against the development of cancer.

polyunsaturated fats: Fats with more than one double bond.

probiotics: Nutrients that provide the body with beneficial flora in the intestines.

resveratrol: An antioxidant and anti-inflammatory found in red wine and red grapes.

rotation diet: A diet for people who suspect they are allergic or have food sensitivities. With rotation, the same food is not eaten days in a row. Usually, after a food is eaten it is not consumed again for three days.

saturated fatty acids: Fats that are completely saturated with hydrogen atoms in their chemical structure. This makes them hard fats.

triglycerides: Neutral fats that combine with proteins in the blood to make lipoproteins.

villi: Hair-like projections from the surface of the intestinal wall lining. Villi increase the surface area of the lining, to allow for the passage of water and nutrients through the intestinal lining into the bloodstream.

xenoestrogens: Foreign substances that have oestrogenic properties. Usually, this term refers to toxic chemicals introduced into the environment that mimic the action of the hormone oestroge

index

index

Enjoyed this? Then visit our website for information on our other *In Essence* titles

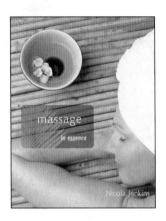

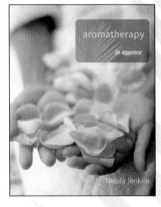

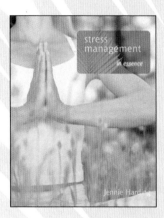

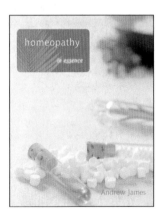

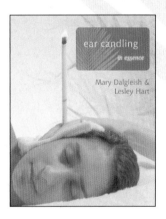

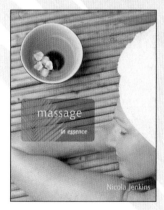

Indulge yourself
www.hoddereducation.co.uk/FE/Therapies